CARNIVORE DIET

Unlocking the Power of Animal-Based

Nutrition

TYLER THOMPSON

1

TABLE OF CONTENTS

Introduction

Welcome to the world of the carnivore diet, where the primal instinct to consume animal foods reigns supreme, and the transformative power of animal-based nutrition is unleashed. In the age of dietary confusion and conflicting nutritional advice, the carnivore diet emerges as a beacon of clarity, offering a simple yet profound approach to optimal health and vitality.

For centuries, humans have relied on animal foods as a primary source of sustenance, fueling our bodies and minds with the nutrient-rich bounty of the natural world. From the hunter-gatherer societies of our ancestors to the modern-day proponents of the carnivore lifestyle, the consumption of meat, fish, and other animal products has been deeply woven into the fabric of human existence.

In recent years, interest in the carnivore diet has surged, driven by compelling anecdotes of remarkable transformations and backed by a growing body of scientific evidence. Contrary to conventional wisdom, which often vilifies animal-based foods, proponents of the carnivore diet assert that these foods hold the key to unlocking our full potential – both physically and mentally.

But what exactly is the carnivore diet, and why has it captured the imagination of so many? At its core, the carnivore diet is a dietary approach that emphasizes the exclusive consumption of animal foods while eschewing plant-based foods altogether. By embracing the nutrient-dense bounty of the animal kingdom, proponents of the carnivore diet believe they can optimize their health, enhance their performance, and reclaim their vitality.

In this book, we embark on a journey to explore the principles, science, and practical application of the carnivore diet. We'll delve into the nutritional composition of animal foods, uncover the scientific research supporting the carnivore diet, and hear from real-life individuals who have experienced its transformative effects firsthand.

But the carnivore diet is more than just a dietary regimen – it's a paradigm shift, challenging conventional beliefs about nutrition and inviting us to reconnect with our ancestral roots. As we embark on this journey together, let us open our minds to the possibilities that lie ahead and embrace the power of animal-based nutrition to unlock our fullest potential.

So join me as we journey into the world of the carnivore diet – a world where the primal instinct to feast on animal foods meets the cutting-edge science of optimal nutrition.

Together, we'll unlock the secrets of the carnivore diet and unleash the power of animal-based nutrition to transform our lives for the better.

Chapter 1

Introduction to the Carnivore Diet

Overview of the carnivore diet philosophy

The carnivore diet is a dietary approach that emphasizes the consumption of animal products while excluding most or all plant-based foods. Advocates of this diet believe that humans evolved as carnivores and that returning to a diet primarily composed of animal foods can improve health and well-being. In this section, we will explore the philosophy behind the carnivore diet, its historical context, scientific rationale, potential benefits and risks, and its implications for individuals and society.

- **Historical Context**

The concept of a carnivore diet is not entirely new; throughout history, various cultures have subsisted primarily on animal foods due to geographical, climatic, or cultural factors. For example, the Inuit people of the Arctic traditionally relied on a diet rich in fish, seal, and other animal products. Similarly, pastoralist societies like the Maasai in Africa have thrived on diets consisting mainly of meat, milk, and blood from cattle.

- **Philosophical Foundations**

The philosophy of the carnivore diet is rooted in several key beliefs:

1. **Evolutionary Adaptation:** Proponents argue that humans evolved as hunters and gatherers, consuming predominantly animal foods for millions of years before the advent of agriculture. They contend that our ancestors' diets were primarily composed of meat, fish, and other animal products, and that our bodies are therefore better adapted to metabolize these foods compared to modern processed foods.

2. **Nutrient Density:** Animal foods are often praised for their high nutrient density, providing essential vitamins, minerals, and amino acids in highly bioavailable forms.

Advocates of the carnivore diet claim that by focusing on nutrient-dense animal foods, individuals can meet their nutritional needs more efficiently than with plant-based diets.

3. **Elimination of Anti-Nutrients:** Plants contain compounds known as anti-nutrients, such as lectins, phytates, and oxalates, which can interfere with nutrient absorption and cause digestive issues in some people. By eliminating plant foods, proponents argue that individuals can avoid these potential negative effects and optimize nutrient absorption.

4. **Potential Health Benefits:** Advocates of the carnivore diet often cite anecdotal reports and emerging research suggesting that it may lead to various health benefits, including weight

loss, improved metabolic health, better mental clarity, and relief from autoimmune conditions and digestive disorders.

- **Scientific Rationale**

While the carnivore diet may seem counterintuitive to conventional dietary recommendations, some scientific principles support its potential efficacy:

✓ **Protein Satiety:** Protein is highly satiating, meaning it can help control appetite and promote feelings of fullness. By prioritizing protein-rich animal foods, individuals may naturally consume fewer calories, potentially leading to weight loss.

✓ **Ketosis and Fat Adaptation:** A strict carnivore diet can induce a state of ketosis, where the body relies primarily on fat for fuel instead of carbohydrates. Ketosis has been associated with various metabolic benefits, including improved insulin sensitivity and fat metabolism.

✓ **Elimination of Trigger Foods:** Many common allergens and sensitivities are found in plant foods, such as gluten in grains or lectins in legumes. By eliminating these potential trigger foods, individuals may experience relief from symptoms associated with food intolerances or autoimmune conditions.

✓ **Nutrient Density of Animal Foods:** Animal foods, particularly organ meats and fatty cuts, are rich sources of essential nutrients such as vitamin B12, heme iron, and omega-3 fatty acids. Prioritizing these nutrient-dense foods can help individuals meet their nutritional needs without relying on supplements or fortified foods.

- **Potential Benefits**

  Advocates of the carnivore diet claim a range of potential benefits, including:

✓ **Weight Loss:** By eliminating carbohydrates and focusing on protein and fat, individuals may naturally reduce calorie intake and achieve weight loss.

✓ **Improved Metabolic Health:** Some research suggests that low-carbohydrate, high-protein diets can improve markers of metabolic health, including blood sugar levels, insulin sensitivity, and lipid profiles.

✓ **Enhanced Mental Clarity:** Supporters of the carnivore diet often report improved cognitive function, focus, and mental clarity, which they attribute to stable blood sugar levels and ketosis.

✓ **Relief from Digestive Issues:** For individuals with gastrointestinal disorders such as irritable bowel syndrome (IBS) or inflammatory bowel disease (IBD), eliminating plant foods may provide relief from symptoms such as bloating, gas, and diarrhea.

- **Potential Risks**

While the carnivore diet may offer certain benefits, it also poses potential risks and challenges:

✓ **Nutritional Deficiencies:** Excluding plant foods can lead to deficiencies in essential nutrients such as fiber, vitamin C, folate, and phytonutrients. Without careful planning, individuals may be at risk of nutrient deficiencies over time.

✓ **Digestive Discomfort:** Some people may experience digestive discomfort, including constipation or diarrhea, when transitioning to a carnivore diet due to changes in fiber intake and gut microbiota.

✓ **Long-Term Health Effects:** The long-term health effects of a carnivore diet are not well understood, particularly regarding cardiovascular health, bone health, and cancer risk. Some studies suggest potential concerns related to increased saturated fat intake and reduced intake of protective phytonutrients.

✓ **Sustainability and Environmental Impact:** From an ethical and environmental perspective, the carnivore diet raises concerns about animal welfare, resource usage, and greenhouse gas emissions associated with livestock production. A diet heavily reliant on animal products may not be sustainable on a global scale.

The carnivore diet represents a radical departure from conventional dietary recommendations, emphasizing the consumption of animal foods while excluding most or all plant-based foods. Proponents of this dietary approach argue that it aligns with human evolutionary history, provides essential nutrients in highly bioavailable forms, and may offer various health benefits, including weight loss, improved metabolic health, and relief from digestive issues. However, the carnivore diet also poses potential risks and challenges, including nutritional deficiencies, digestive discomfort, and concerns about long-term health effects and environmental sustainability. As with any dietary approach, individuals considering the carnivore diet should carefully weigh its potential benefits and risks and consult with healthcare professionals to ensure nutritional adequacy and overall health. Further research is needed to better understand the effects of the carnivore diet on human health and its implications for individuals and society.

Customizing the diet based on individual needs and goals

Customizing the carnivore diet based on individual needs and goals involves tailoring this dietary approach to suit an individual's unique preferences, health status, fitness goals, and lifestyle. While the carnivore diet is often portrayed as a strict regimen focused solely on animal products, there is room for flexibility and personalization within this framework. In this section, we will explore various factors to consider when customizing the carnivore diet, including protein intake, food choices, nutrient density, supplementation, exercise, and long-term sustainability.

The carnivore diet emphasizes the consumption of animal foods while excluding most or all plant-based foods. Commonly included foods are meat, fish, poultry, eggs, and certain dairy products such as cheese and butter. Advocates of the carnivore diet often recommend prioritizing nutrient-dense animal foods, including organ meats, fatty cuts of meat, and bone broth, while avoiding processed meats and high-carbohydrate dairy products.

- **Factors to Consider When Customizing**

1. Protein Intake

Protein is a crucial macronutrient for muscle growth, repair, and overall health. When customizing the carnivore diet, individuals should consider their protein needs based on factors such as age, gender, body composition, activity level, and fitness goals. Athletes and those engaging in intense physical activity may require higher protein intake to support muscle recovery and performance. Including a variety of protein sources, such as beef, chicken, fish, and eggs, can help ensure adequate amino acid intake.

2. Food Choices

While animal foods form the foundation of the carnivore diet, there is flexibility in choosing which types of animal products to include based on personal preference, availability, and dietary restrictions. Some individuals may prefer fatty cuts of meat for their higher calorie content and flavor, while others may prioritize leaner protein sources. Including a variety of animal foods, such as red meat, poultry, seafood, and organ meats, can provide a broad spectrum of nutrients and prevent dietary monotony.

3. Nutrient Density

Nutrient density refers to the concentration of essential nutrients per calorie in a food. When customizing the carnivore diet, individuals should prioritize nutrient-dense animal foods to meet their nutritional needs effectively. Organ meats, such as liver, kidney, and heart, are particularly rich sources of vitamins, minerals, and antioxidants. Including a variety of animal foods in the diet ensures a diverse array of nutrients and minimizes the risk of nutrient deficiencies.

4. Supplementation

While the carnivore diet can provide many essential nutrients, certain micronutrients may be lacking or insufficiently represented in animal foods alone. Individuals following a carnivore diet may consider supplementation to address potential nutrient gaps. Common supplements include vitamin D, omega-3 fatty acids, magnesium, and electrolytes. Consulting with a healthcare professional or registered dietitian can help determine appropriate supplementation based on individual needs and goals.

5. Exercise

Physical activity plays a crucial role in overall health and fitness, regardless of dietary approach. When customizing the carnivore diet, individuals should consider their exercise routine and energy expenditure to ensure adequate fueling and recovery. Consuming sufficient protein and calories is essential for supporting muscle growth, repair, and performance. Pre- and post-workout nutrition, including protein-rich meals or snacks, can help optimize exercise performance and recovery on the carnivore diet.

6. Long-Term Sustainability

Sustainability is a key consideration when adopting any dietary approach. While the carnivore diet may offer certain benefits in the short term, its long-term sustainability depends on factors such as nutrient adequacy, dietary variety, and adherence. Individuals should assess whether the carnivore diet aligns with their lifestyle, cultural preferences, ethical beliefs, and environmental values.

Experimenting with different foods, recipes, and meal plans can help enhance the sustainability and enjoyment of the carnivore diet over time.

- **Practical Tips for Customizing the Carnivore Diet**

✓ **Experiment with Different Foods:** Explore a variety of animal foods, including different cuts of meat, fish, poultry, and organ meats, to find what works best for you in terms of taste, texture, and nutritional profile.

✓ **Monitor Nutrient Intake:** Use food tracking apps or consult with a registered dietitian to ensure you are meeting your nutritional needs on the carnivore diet, paying particular attention to protein, vitamins, and minerals.

- ✓ **Include Fatty Cuts of Meat:** Incorporate fatty cuts of meat, such as ribeye steak, pork belly, and salmon, to increase calorie intake and provide essential fatty acids for optimal health.

- ✓ **Experiment with Cooking Methods:** Explore different cooking methods, such as grilling, roasting, braising, and stewing, to enhance the flavor and texture of animal foods and prevent dietary monotony.

- ✓ **Stay Hydrated:** Drink plenty of water throughout the day to stay hydrated, especially if you are consuming higher amounts of protein, which can increase water needs.

- ✓ **Listen to Your Body:** Pay attention to hunger cues, energy levels, and digestive health to determine how the carnivore diet is affecting your overall well-being, and make adjustments as needed.

Customizing the carnivore diet based on individual needs and goals involves tailoring this dietary approach to suit preferences, health status, fitness goals, and lifestyle. By considering factors such as protein intake, food choices, nutrient density, supplementation, exercise, and long-term sustainability, individuals can optimize the carnivore diet to meet their unique nutritional needs effectively. Experimenting with different foods, monitoring nutrient intake, and listening to your body's signals can help enhance the enjoyment, effectiveness, and sustainability of the carnivore diet over time. As with any dietary approach, it's essential to consult with healthcare professionals or registered dietitians to ensure nutritional adequacy and overall health.

Selecting quality animal foods and sourcing options

Selecting high-quality animal foods and sourcing options is paramount for individuals adhering to the carnivore diet. The quality of animal products can significantly impact nutritional content, taste, and overall health outcomes. In this section, we will explore the importance of selecting quality animal foods, factors to consider when sourcing animal products, and various options for obtaining high-quality meat, fish, poultry, eggs, and dairy products on the carnivore diet.

- **Importance of Quality Animal Foods:**

Quality animal foods provide essential nutrients such as protein, vitamins, minerals, and healthy fats necessary for optimal health and well-being. Factors such as animal diet, farming practices, and processing methods can influence the nutritional content and safety of animal products. Selecting high-quality animal foods ensures greater nutrient density, better taste, and reduced exposure to harmful substances such as antibiotics, hormones, and pesticides.

- **Factors to Consider When Sourcing Animal Products**

1. Animal Diet

The diet of the animals directly influences the nutritional composition of their meat, eggs, and dairy products. Animals raised on pasture or grass-fed diets tend to produce meat and dairy products higher in omega-3 fatty acids, conjugated linoleic acid (CLA), and vitamins compared to conventionally raised animals fed grain-based diets. Look for products labeled "grass-fed," "pasture-raised," or "free-range" to ensure higher nutrient content and better animal welfare.

2. Farming Practices

The farming practices employed by producers can impact animal health, environmental sustainability, and product quality. Choose products from farms and producers committed to ethical and sustainable farming practices, such as rotational grazing, humane animal treatment, and minimal use of antibiotics and synthetic hormones. Certification programs like Animal Welfare Approved (AWA), Certified Humane, and Organic ensure higher standards of animal welfare and environmental stewardship.

3. Processing Methods

The processing methods used for animal products can affect their taste, texture, and safety. Opt for minimally processed meats and dairy products without added preservatives, fillers, or artificial ingredients. Choose products from reputable producers and butcher shops known for their commitment to quality and food safety standards.

4. Environmental Impact

Consider the environmental impact of animal agriculture when sourcing animal products. Look for products from producers implementing sustainable farming practices, such as regenerative agriculture, carbon sequestration, and biodiversity conservation. Choosing locally sourced products reduces carbon emissions associated with transportation and supports local economies.

5. Budget and Affordability

While prioritizing quality is essential, consider your budget and affordability when sourcing animal products. Look for cost-effective options such as buying in bulk, joining meat subscription services, or purchasing directly from local farmers and producers. Consider investing in higher-quality products for staple items like meat and eggs while opting for more affordable options for occasional treats or supplements.

- **Options for Sourcing Quality Animal Foods**

1. Local Farms and Farmers' Markets

Local farms and farmers' markets offer a direct and transparent source of high-quality animal products. Look for farms and producers in your area that specialize in pasture-raised meats, free-range eggs, and artisanal dairy products. Building relationships with local farmers allows you to learn about their farming practices, ask questions, and support the local food system.

2. Online Retailers and Meat Subscription Services

Online retailers and meat subscription services provide convenient access to a wide selection of high-quality animal products. Look for reputable online retailers and subscription services that prioritize quality, sustainability, and customer satisfaction. Many services offer customizable meat boxes, specialty cuts, and curated selections tailored to individual preferences and dietary needs.

3. Specialty Butcher Shops and Delis

Specialty butcher shops and delis often source their meat from local farms and producers known for their commitment to quality and sustainability. Visit butcher shops and delis in your area that specialize in grass-fed, pasture-raised, or organic meats. Build a relationship with your butcher to receive personalized recommendations, cooking tips, and updates on seasonal offerings.

4. Community Supported Agriculture (CSA) Programs

Community Supported Agriculture (CSA) programs allow consumers to purchase shares of a farm's harvest in advance, typically receiving a weekly or monthly supply of seasonal produce, meat, eggs, and dairy products. Joining a CSA program connects you directly with local farmers and provides a reliable source of fresh, seasonal, and sustainably grown foods.

5. Wild-Caught Seafood Suppliers

When sourcing seafood, prioritize wild-caught options over farm-raised varieties whenever possible. Look for reputable suppliers and retailers specializing in sustainably sourced seafood, such as certified fisheries and seafood watch programs. Consider purchasing directly from fishermen's cooperatives, seafood markets, or online retailers offering a wide selection of wild-caught fish and shellfish.

6. Home Production

For individuals with the necessary space, resources, and expertise, home production of animal foods is an option. Consider raising backyard chickens for fresh eggs, keeping small livestock such as rabbits or goats for meat and dairy products, or hunting and fishing for wild game. Home production allows you to have greater control over the quality, safety, and sustainability of your animal products.

Selecting high-quality animal foods and sourcing options is essential for individuals following the carnivore diet to ensure optimal nutrition, taste, and overall health outcomes. By considering factors such as animal diet, farming practices, processing methods, environmental impact, and budget, individuals can make informed choices when purchasing meat, fish, poultry, eggs, and dairy products. Exploring various sourcing options, including local farms, online retailers, specialty butcher shops, community-supported agriculture programs, and home production, allows individuals to access a diverse array of high-quality animal foods tailored to their preferences and dietary needs. Prioritizing quality, sustainability, and transparency in sourcing animal products contributes to the well-being of both consumers and the environment, supporting a healthier and more ethical food system.

Creating balanced meals and optimizing nutrient intake

Creating balanced meals and optimizing nutrient intake is essential for individuals following any dietary approach, including the carnivore diet. While the carnivore diet primarily focuses on animal products, it's still crucial to ensure adequate intake of essential nutrients to support overall health and well-being. In this section, we will explore strategies for creating balanced meals on the carnivore diet, factors to consider when optimizing nutrient intake, and practical tips for achieving nutritional adequacy while prioritizing animal foods.

- **Importance of Balanced Meals**

Balanced meals provide a combination of macronutrients, micronutrients, and other essential compounds necessary for optimal health and function. On the carnivore diet, creating balanced meals involves incorporating a variety of animal foods to ensure adequate intake of protein, healthy fats, vitamins, and minerals. Balancing nutrient intake promotes satiety, supports energy levels, and helps prevent nutrient deficiencies and imbalances.

- **Macronutrient Ratios on the Carnivore Diet**

The macronutrient ratios on the carnivore diet typically consist of:

Protein: A cornerstone of the carnivore diet, protein is essential for muscle growth, repair, and overall health. Aim to include protein-rich animal foods such as meat, fish, poultry, and eggs in each meal to meet your protein needs.

Fat: Fat provides a concentrated source of energy and essential fatty acids on the carnivore diet. Include fatty cuts of meat, organ meats, and high-fat dairy products to ensure an adequate intake of healthy fats.

Carbohydrates: While the carnivore diet is inherently low in carbohydrates, some individuals may include small amounts of carbohydrates from dairy products or incidental sources. However, carbohydrates are typically minimized on the carnivore diet, with the focus primarily on protein and fat.

- **Optimizing Nutrient Intake**

1. Prioritize Nutrient-Dense Foods

Choose nutrient-dense animal foods that provide a wide range of vitamins, minerals, and other essential nutrients. Include a variety of meats, poultry, fish, organ meats, eggs, and dairy products in your diet to ensure a diverse array of nutrients.

2. Include Organ Meats

Organ meats, such as liver, kidney, heart, and brain, are nutritional powerhouses rich in vitamins, minerals, and antioxidants. Incorporate organ meats into your meals regularly to boost your intake of essential nutrients like vitamin A, vitamin B12, iron, and zinc.

3. Eat Nose-to-Tail

Embrace the nose-to-tail approach by consuming all parts of the animal, including muscle meats, organs, bones, and connective tissues. Each part of the animal offers a unique nutritional profile, contributing to overall nutrient adequacy and health benefits.

4. Include Bone Broth

Bone broth is a nutrient-rich beverage made by simmering animal bones and connective tissues in water. It provides a concentrated source of collagen, amino acids, minerals, and other beneficial compounds. Incorporate bone broth into your meals as a flavorful base for soups, stews, and sauces.

5. Choose Quality Sources

Select high-quality animal products from reputable sources that prioritize ethical and sustainable farming practices. Look for grass-fed and pasture-raised meats, wild-caught fish, organic poultry, and free-range eggs to ensure higher nutrient content and better animal welfare.

6. Monitor Nutrient Intake

Track your nutrient intake using food diary apps or consult with a registered dietitian to ensure you're meeting your nutritional needs on the carnivore diet. Pay attention to essential nutrients like protein, vitamins (especially vitamin B12, vitamin D, and vitamin A), minerals (such as iron, zinc, and magnesium), and omega-3 fatty acids.

- **Practical Tips for Balanced Meals**

1. Include a Variety of Animal Foods

Aim to include a variety of animal foods in each meal to ensure a broad spectrum of nutrients. Mix and match different cuts of meat, poultry, fish, and organ meats to add variety and flavor to your meals.

2. Balance Protein and Fat Intake

Balance your protein and fat intake to meet your energy needs and promote satiety. Include fatty cuts of meat, skin-on poultry, and high-fat dairy products to increase fat intake if needed.

3. Incorporate Eggs

Eggs are a versatile and nutritious addition to the carnivore diet, providing high-quality protein, healthy fats, vitamins, and minerals.

Include whole eggs or egg yolks in your meals to boost nutrient intake and add variety.

4. Season with Herbs and Spices

While the carnivore diet primarily focuses on animal foods, you can enhance flavor and enjoyment by seasoning your meals with herbs, spices, and condiments. Choose natural seasonings like salt, pepper, garlic, onion powder, and fresh herbs to add depth of flavor without adding carbohydrates.

5. Experiment with Cooking Methods

Explore different cooking methods, such as grilling, roasting, braising, and stewing, to enhance the taste and texture of animal foods.

Experiment with cooking techniques and recipes to keep meals exciting and satisfying.

6. Include Fermented Foods

Fermented foods such as cheese, yogurt, and kefir can provide additional nutrients and beneficial bacteria for gut health. Include small amounts of fermented dairy products in your meals to support digestion and immune function.

Creating balanced meals and optimizing nutrient intake on the carnivore diet involves incorporating a variety of high-quality animal foods to ensure adequate protein, fat, vitamins, and minerals. Prioritizing nutrient-dense foods such as organ meats, bone broth, and eggs, choosing quality sources from ethical and sustainable producers, and monitoring nutrient intake are essential strategies for achieving nutritional adequacy. By following practical tips for balanced meals, including a variety of animal foods, balancing protein and fat intake, incorporating eggs and seasoning with herbs and spices, individuals can optimize their nutrient intake and support overall health and well-being on the carnivore diet. As with any dietary approach, it's essential to listen to your body, experiment with different foods and cooking methods, and seek guidance from healthcare professionals or registered dietitians to ensure nutritional adequacy and long-term success.

Chapter 2

Understanding Animal-Based Nutrition

Nutritional composition of animal foods

The nutritional composition of animal foods is a complex and multifaceted topic that encompasses a wide range of nutrients essential for human health. Animal foods, including meat, poultry, fish, eggs, and dairy products, have long been a significant part of human diets across cultures and civilizations. They provide a rich source of protein, essential fatty acids, vitamins, and minerals, which are crucial for various physiological functions and overall well-being. In this discussion, we'll delve into the nutritional composition of different types of animal foods, their health benefits, and considerations regarding consumption.

1. Protein

Animal foods are renowned for their high-quality protein content, which contains all essential amino acids required by the human body. Protein is essential for muscle growth and repair, immune function, hormone production, and enzyme activity. Meats such as beef, poultry, pork, and lamb are particularly rich in protein, with varying levels of fat content depending on the cut and type of meat.

2. Fats

Animal foods provide various types of fats, including saturated fats, monounsaturated fats, and polyunsaturated fats. While excessive consumption of saturated fats has been associated with increased risk of cardiovascular disease, certain animal foods like fatty fish contain omega-3 fatty acids, which have cardioprotective effects. Eggs and dairy products also contain a mix of fats, with some controversy surrounding their impact on health, particularly regarding cholesterol levels.

3. Vitamins

Animal foods are significant sources of several vitamins essential for health. For example, vitamin B12, primarily found in meat, fish, eggs, and dairy, is crucial for nerve function and the formation of red blood cells. Other B vitamins, including riboflavin, niacin, and B6, are also abundant in animal foods and play roles in energy metabolism and cell function. Additionally, animal foods provide vitamin A, important for vision, immune function, and skin health, primarily in the form of retinol found in liver and dairy products.

4. Minerals

Animal foods are rich sources of various minerals vital for maintaining health. Iron, primarily found in red meat, poultry, and fish, is essential for oxygen transport in the blood and the functioning of enzymes involved in energy metabolism. Zinc, abundant in meat and shellfish, is crucial for immune function, wound healing, and DNA synthesis. Additionally, animal foods provide significant amounts of calcium, phosphorus, magnesium, and selenium, important for bone health, muscle function, and antioxidant defense mechanisms.

5. Other Nutrients

In addition to protein, fats, vitamins, and minerals, animal foods contain other bioactive compounds with potential health benefits. For example, creatine, predominantly found in meat, is involved in energy metabolism and may enhance athletic performance. Taurine, abundant in seafood and meat, plays roles in bile salt formation, antioxidant defense, and cardiovascular health. Moreover, certain animal foods like bone broth contain collagen, gelatin, and other compounds beneficial for joint health and gut integrity.

Health Considerations

While animal foods offer a rich source of essential nutrients, their consumption should be part of a balanced diet, considering individual health needs and preferences. Excessive intake of red and processed meats has been associated with an increased risk of chronic diseases such as cardiovascular disease, certain cancers, and type 2 diabetes. Therefore, it's essential to choose lean cuts of meat, minimize processed meat consumption, and focus on a variety of animal and plant-based foods to optimize nutrient intake and overall health.

Furthermore, concerns about animal welfare, environmental sustainability, and ethical considerations have led many individuals to explore plant-based alternatives or adopt flexitarian, vegetarian, or vegan diets. Plant-based sources of protein, such as legumes, tofu, tempeh, and nuts, can provide adequate nutrition when consumed in sufficient quantities and variety. However, careful attention must be paid to ensure adequate intake of certain nutrients commonly found in animal foods, such as vitamin B12, iron, zinc, and omega-3 fatty acids, through fortified foods or supplements.

The nutritional composition of animal foods encompasses a diverse array of nutrients essential for human health, including protein, fats, vitamins, minerals, and other bioactive compounds. While animal foods can contribute to a well-balanced diet, their consumption should be moderated, with consideration given to individual health needs, environmental sustainability, and ethical concerns. Incorporating a variety of animal and plant-based foods into one's diet can help optimize nutrient intake and promote overall health and well-being.

Exploring bioavailability and nutrient density

The carnivore diet, characterized by the exclusive consumption of animal-derived foods, has gained popularity in recent years as a dietary approach claimed to offer various health benefits. Advocates of the carnivore diet argue that eliminating plant-based foods can improve digestion, reduce inflammation, and promote weight loss. However, the nutritional adequacy, bioavailability, and long-term health implications of such a diet remain subjects of debate and scrutiny. In this discussion, we will explore the bioavailability and nutrient density of the carnivore diet, considering its potential benefits and limitations.

1. Bioavailability of Nutrients

Bioavailability refers to the extent and rate at which nutrients from food are absorbed and utilized by the body. Animal-derived foods are generally rich sources of highly bioavailable nutrients, including protein, fats, vitamins, and minerals. The absence of anti-nutrients, such as phytates and oxalates found in plant foods, may enhance the absorption of certain nutrients in the carnivore diet.

2. Nutrient Density

Nutrient density refers to the concentration of essential nutrients per calorie in a given food. Animal-derived foods are often highly nutrient-dense, providing a wide array of essential nutrients in relatively small serving sizes. However, the nutrient density of the carnivore diet may vary depending on the types of animal foods consumed and their preparation methods.

Lean vs. Fatty Cuts

Choosing lean cuts of meat, poultry, and fish can help maximize nutrient density while minimizing calorie and fat intake. Lean meats provide high-quality protein, vitamins, and minerals with fewer calories and less saturated fat compared to fatty cuts. However, including moderate amounts of fatty cuts or incorporating sources of healthy fats such as fatty fish, eggs, and dairy products can enhance the nutrient density of the carnivore diet and promote satiety.

Organ Meats

Organ meats, such as liver, heart, kidneys, and tongue, are nutritional powerhouses packed with vitamins, minerals, and bioactive compounds. Liver, in particular, is one of the most nutrient-dense foods, containing high levels of vitamin A, B vitamins, iron, zinc, and other essential nutrients. Incorporating organ meats into the carnivore diet can significantly boost its nutrient density and provide a diverse array of essential nutrients not found in muscle meats alone.

Bone Broth

Bone broth, made by simmering animal bones and connective tissue, is rich in collagen, gelatin, and other compounds beneficial for joint health, gut integrity, and skin health. Bone broth is also a source of minerals such as calcium, magnesium, and phosphorus, which are leached from the bones during the cooking process. Including bone broth in the carnivore diet can enhance its nutrient density and provide additional health benefits.

3. Considerations and Limitations

While the carnivore diet may offer some benefits in terms of nutrient bioavailability and density, it also has several considerations and limitations that should be taken into account.

Nutrient Imbalance

Eliminating plant-based foods from the diet may lead to nutrient imbalances and deficiencies if not carefully planned. Certain vitamins and minerals, such as vitamin C, fiber, and phytonutrients, are predominantly found in plant foods and may be lacking in a carnivore diet. Adequate intake of vitamin C can be obtained from organ meats and certain animal-derived foods, but supplementation may be necessary for some individuals.

Fiber Intake

The carnivore diet is devoid of dietary fiber, which plays crucial roles in digestive health, satiety, and blood sugar regulation. While some proponents argue that fiber is not essential for human health and may even cause digestive issues in some individuals, others emphasize the importance of including fiber-rich foods to support gut microbiota diversity and overall well-being.

Long-Term Health Effects:

The long-term health effects of the carnivore diet are not well-understood, and further research is needed to evaluate its safety and efficacy over extended periods. While some individuals may experience short-term benefits such as weight loss, improved digestion, and increased energy levels on a carnivore diet, the potential risks of nutrient deficiencies, cardiovascular disease, and other health complications should be carefully considered.

Environmental and Ethical Concerns

The exclusive consumption of animal-derived foods in the carnivore diet raises environmental and ethical concerns related to animal welfare, greenhouse gas emissions, and sustainable food production. Large-scale livestock farming contributes to deforestation, habitat destruction, and water pollution, while also raising ethical questions about the treatment of animals raised for food.

The carnivore diet emphasizes the consumption of animal-derived foods while excluding plant-based foods. While animal foods are rich sources of highly bioavailable nutrients and can be highly nutrient-dense, the carnivore diet may pose challenges in terms of nutrient balance, fiber intake, and long-term health effects. Individuals considering a carnivore diet should carefully weigh the potential benefits and limitations, seek guidance from healthcare professionals or registered dietitians, and ensure adequate nutrient intake through a varied and balanced diet. Additionally, environmental and ethical considerations should be taken into account when making dietary choices to promote sustainability and ethical food practices.

Debunking common misconceptions about animal-based diets

Debunking common misconceptions about animal-based diets requires a comprehensive examination of the scientific evidence surrounding the consumption of animal-derived foods and their impact on health, the environment, and ethical considerations. While animal-based diets have been a significant part of human nutrition for centuries, they are often subject to various misconceptions and myths. In this discussion, we will explore and debunk some of the most prevalent misconceptions about animal-based diets.

1. Animal-Based Diets Are Unhealthy

One of the most persistent misconceptions is that animal-based diets are inherently unhealthy and contribute to various chronic diseases. While excessive consumption of certain animal-derived foods, particularly processed meats and fatty cuts of red meat, has been associated with increased risk of cardiovascular disease, type 2 diabetes, and certain cancers, moderate intake of lean sources of protein and healthy fats can be part of a balanced diet.

Debunking the Myth

Numerous studies have demonstrated that including lean cuts of meat, poultry, fish, eggs, and dairy products as part of a balanced diet can provide essential nutrients such as high-quality protein, vitamins (e.g., B12, riboflavin, niacin), minerals (e.g., iron, zinc, calcium), and omega-3 fatty acids, which are crucial for overall health. Additionally, evidence suggests that the Mediterranean diet, which includes moderate consumption of animal-derived foods along with plenty of fruits, vegetables, whole grains, and healthy fats, is associated with reduced risk of chronic diseases and improved longevity.

2. Animal-Based Diets Are Not Sustainable

Another common misconception is that animal-based diets are environmentally unsustainable due to their impact on land use, water consumption, greenhouse gas emissions, and biodiversity loss. The industrial livestock industry, characterized by large-scale confinement operations and intensive feed production, has been criticized for its environmental footprint and contribution to climate change.

Debunking the Myth

While industrial livestock farming does pose significant environmental challenges, not all animal-based diets are inherently unsustainable. Sustainable animal agriculture practices, such as rotational grazing, regenerative farming, and agroecology, can help minimize environmental impact, promote soil health, enhance biodiversity, and sequester carbon. Moreover, integrating animal husbandry with crop production can create synergies and closed-loop systems that reduce waste and improve resource efficiency.

3. Animal-Based Diets Are Cruel to Animals

Many people believe that animal-based diets inherently involve cruelty to animals, particularly in industrial farming operations where animals are confined in overcrowded and unsanitary conditions, subjected to routine use of antibiotics and growth hormones, and deprived of natural behaviors.

Debunking the Myth

While industrial farming practices raise legitimate concerns about animal welfare, not all animal-based diets rely on cruel treatment of animals. Ethical animal husbandry practices, such as pasture-raised, free-range, and organic farming, prioritize animal welfare, provide access to outdoor spaces, and allow animals to express natural behaviors. Additionally, small-scale and family-owned farms often prioritize humane treatment of animals and maintain closer relationships between farmers and livestock.

4. Animal-Based Diets Are Not Ethical

Some people argue that consuming animal-derived foods is unethical due to concerns about animal welfare, environmental degradation, and global food inequities. They advocate for plant-based diets or veganism as more ethical alternatives that minimize harm to animals, the environment, and human health.

Debunking the Myth

The ethics of consuming animal-derived foods are complex and multifaceted, and individual perspectives may vary based on cultural, religious, and personal beliefs. While reducing meat consumption and incorporating more plant-based foods into the diet can have environmental and ethical benefits, ethical omnivorism is another approach that emphasizes responsible sourcing, transparency, and conscious consumption of animal-derived foods. Supporting local and sustainable food systems, choosing humanely raised and ethically sourced animal products, and reducing food waste can align with ethical principles while still including animal-based foods in the diet.

5. Animal-Based Diets Are Incompatible With Environmental Conservation

Another misconception is that consuming animal-derived foods is incompatible with environmental conservation and efforts to mitigate climate change. Some argue that transitioning to plant-based diets or veganism is necessary to reduce greenhouse gas emissions, conserve natural resources, and protect ecosystems.

Debunking the Myth

While reducing meat consumption and shifting towards plant-based diets can reduce environmental impact, not all animal-based diets are inherently detrimental to environmental conservation. Sustainable animal agriculture practices, such as rotational grazing, silvopasture, and holistic land management, can enhance ecosystem health, restore degraded lands, and promote carbon sequestration. Moreover, integrating livestock into regenerative agricultural systems can contribute to biodiversity conservation, soil fertility, and watershed protection.

Debunking common misconceptions about animal-based diets requires a nuanced understanding of the scientific evidence, ethical considerations, and environmental implications surrounding the consumption of animal-derived foods. While animal-based diets have been subject to criticism and scrutiny, they can be part of a healthy, sustainable, and ethical diet when sourced responsibly and consumed mindfully. By addressing misconceptions and promoting informed decision-making, we can foster a more balanced and inclusive dialogue about

dietary choices that prioritize human health,

animal welfare, environmental sustainability,

and ethical considerations.

Chapter 3

The Science Behind the Carnivore Diet

Research and studies supporting the carnivore diet

Advocates of the carnivore diet claim various health benefits, including weight loss, improved mental clarity, increased energy levels, and relief from certain health conditions such as autoimmune disorders and digestive issues. While this dietary approach has gained popularity in recent years, it remains controversial due to its deviation from conventional dietary recommendations promoting a balanced intake of fruits, vegetables, whole grains, and other plant-based foods. In this part, we will explore the research and studies supporting the carnivore diet, as well as its potential benefits and drawbacks.

- **Evolutionary Perspective and Anthropological Evidence**

Proponents of the carnivore diet often cite evolutionary biology and anthropological evidence to support their claims. They argue that humans have evolved as apex predators and that animal foods were a primary source of nutrition for our ancestors. Research into the diets of hunter-gatherer societies, such as the Inuit people of the Arctic and the Maasai tribe of East Africa, provides examples of populations that have thrived on predominantly animal-based diets. Studies have shown that these populations exhibited excellent health markers despite consuming minimal plant foods, challenging the notion that a varied diet is necessary for optimal health.

- **Nutrient Density and Bioavailability**

Animal foods are highly nutrient-dense, containing essential vitamins, minerals, and amino acids in easily absorbable forms. Meat is a complete protein source, providing all the essential amino acids required for muscle growth, repair, and various physiological functions. Additionally, animal foods are rich in nutrients such as vitamin B12, iron, zinc, and omega-3 fatty acids, which are crucial for overall health and well-being. Compared to plant-based sources of nutrients, animal foods often have higher bioavailability, meaning that the body can absorb and utilize these nutrients more efficiently.

- **Potential Health Benefits**

Several studies and anecdotal reports suggest that the carnivore diet may offer several health benefits:

Weight Loss: By eliminating carbohydrates and focusing on protein and fat, the carnivore diet may promote weight loss through increased satiety and reduced calorie intake.

Some studies have shown that low-carbohydrate, high-protein diets can lead to greater weight loss compared to traditional low-fat diets.

Improved Metabolic Health: The carnivore diet may improve markers of metabolic health, such as blood glucose levels, insulin sensitivity, and lipid profiles. By reducing carbohydrate intake, the diet may help regulate blood sugar levels and lower triglyceride levels, which are risk factors for metabolic syndrome and cardiovascular disease.

Reduced Inflammation: Certain inflammatory conditions, such as arthritis, autoimmune disorders, and gastrointestinal issues, may improve on a carnivore diet due to the elimination of potentially inflammatory plant foods. Some individuals report relief from symptoms such as joint pain, bloating, and digestive discomfort after adopting a carnivore diet.

Mental Clarity and Cognitive Function: Advocates of the carnivore diet often report improved mental clarity, focus, and cognitive function. While scientific evidence is limited, some studies suggest that ketogenic diets, which share similarities with the carnivore diet in terms of carbohydrate restriction, may have neuroprotective effects and improve cognitive function in certain populations.

Simplicity and Convenience: The carnivore diet offers simplicity and convenience in meal planning and preparation, as it eliminates the need to cook or consume a wide variety of foods. This aspect may be appealing to individuals who prefer straightforward dietary guidelines and minimal food choices.

Drawbacks and Considerations

Despite the potential benefits, the carnivore diet also has several drawbacks and considerations:

✓ **Nutritional Deficiencies:** A strict carnivore diet may lack certain nutrients found in plant-based foods, such as fiber, vitamin C, phytonutrients, and antioxidants. Long-term adherence to the diet without proper supplementation or careful food selection could lead to nutrient deficiencies and health complications.

✓ **Digestive Issues:** Some individuals may experience digestive discomfort, constipation, or other gastrointestinal issues when transitioning to a carnivore diet, particularly if they abruptly eliminate fiber-rich plant foods from their diet. It may take time for the gut microbiota to adapt to a lower-fiber diet, potentially leading to temporary digestive disturbances.

✓ **Potential Health Risks:** Long-term adherence to a carnivore diet may pose certain health risks, including increased risk of heart disease, certain cancers, and kidney stones. High intake of saturated fat and cholesterol from animal foods could elevate cholesterol levels and contribute to cardiovascular problems, particularly in individuals with preexisting risk factors.

✓ **Sustainability and Environmental Impact:** From a sustainability standpoint, the carnivore diet may raise concerns due to its reliance on animal agriculture, which has significant environmental implications, including greenhouse gas emissions, land use, and water consumption. Promoting large-scale consumption of animal products may not be environmentally sustainable in the long term.

✓ **Individual Variability:** It's essential to recognize that not everyone will respond the same way to a carnivore diet. Individual factors such as genetics, metabolic health, activity level, and personal preferences can influence how the body reacts to dietary changes. What works for one person may not work for another, and it's crucial to listen to your body and adjust your diet accordingly.

- **Research Limitations and Areas for Further Study**

While there is growing interest in the carnivore diet, research on its long-term health effects and safety is limited. Most studies examining low-carbohydrate or high-protein diets have focused on short-term outcomes, and more research is needed to understand the potential risks and benefits of a carnivore diet over the long term. Additionally, the majority of existing studies have been observational or anecdotal in nature, lacking rigorous scientific controls and randomized clinical trials. Future research should aim to address these limitations by conducting well-designed studies with larger sample sizes and longer follow-up periods.

The carnivore diet is a dietary approach that emphasizes the consumption of animal foods while excluding most plant-based foods. Proponents of the diet claim various health benefits, including weight loss, improved metabolic health, reduced inflammation, and enhanced cognitive function. While there is some evidence to support these claims, research on the carnivore diet remains limited, and the long-term health effects and safety of the diet are not well understood. Individuals considering the carnivore diet should carefully weigh the potential benefits and drawbacks, consult with healthcare professionals, and make informed decisions based on their individual health needs and preferences. Further research is needed to elucidate the effects of the carnivore diet on health outcomes and to better understand its role in the context of overall dietary patterns and lifestyle factors.

Impact on metabolic health, weight management, and disease prevention

In this part, we will explore the impact of the carnivore diet on metabolic health, weight management, and disease prevention, drawing upon available evidence and research findings.

- **Metabolic Health**

Metabolic health refers to the state of various physiological processes involved in energy metabolism, glucose regulation, lipid metabolism, and insulin sensitivity. The carnivore diet's emphasis on animal foods and exclusion of carbohydrates may influence metabolic parameters in several ways:

Improved Insulin Sensitivity: By minimizing carbohydrate intake, the carnivore diet may improve insulin sensitivity and reduce insulin resistance, leading to better blood sugar control and lower fasting insulin levels. Some studies have shown that low-carbohydrate diets can lead to significant improvements in insulin sensitivity, particularly in individuals with insulin resistance or type 2 diabetes.

Stable Blood Glucose Levels: The carnivore diet's reliance on protein and fat for energy may help stabilize blood glucose levels, preventing the large fluctuations commonly associated with high-carbohydrate meals. This may be beneficial for individuals with diabetes or prediabetes, as well as those seeking to optimize their metabolic health.

Reduced Risk of Metabolic Syndrome:
Metabolic syndrome is a cluster of conditions, including obesity, high blood pressure, elevated blood sugar levels, and abnormal lipid levels, that increase the risk of cardiovascular disease and type 2 diabetes. Some research suggests that low-carbohydrate diets, such as the carnivore diet, may help reduce the risk of metabolic syndrome by addressing underlying metabolic dysfunctions.

Potential Anti-inflammatory Effects:
Chronic inflammation plays a significant role in the development of metabolic disorders such as insulin resistance and obesity. Animal foods, particularly fatty fish, are rich in omega-3 fatty acids, which possess anti-inflammatory

properties. By prioritizing animal foods and minimizing pro-inflammatory plant foods, the carnivore diet may help reduce systemic inflammation and improve metabolic health.

- **Weight Management**

Weight management encompasses various strategies aimed at achieving and maintaining a healthy body weight. The carnivore diet's focus on protein and fat while eliminating carbohydrates may influence weight loss and body composition through several mechanisms:

Increased Satiety: Protein and fat are highly satiating macronutrients that can help regulate appetite and reduce overall calorie intake. By prioritizing animal foods rich in protein and healthy fats, the carnivore diet may promote feelings of fullness and satisfaction, making it easier for individuals to adhere to a calorie-restricted diet and achieve weight loss goals.

Enhanced Fat Oxidation: The ketogenic nature of the carnivore diet, characterized by the production of ketone bodies from fat metabolism, may enhance fat oxidation and promote weight loss. By restricting carbohydrate intake and depleting glycogen stores, the body switches to using fat as its primary fuel source, leading to increased fat burning and weight loss.

Preservation of Lean Body Mass: Unlike traditional low-calorie diets that often lead to loss of lean muscle mass along with fat mass, the high protein content of the carnivore diet may help preserve lean body mass during weight loss. Adequate protein intake is essential for maintaining muscle mass, supporting metabolic rate, and promoting fat loss while minimizing muscle loss.

Reduction in Water Weight: Carbohydrates stored in the body as glycogen are accompanied by water molecules. By depleting glycogen stores through carbohydrate restriction, the carnivore diet may lead to rapid initial weight loss due to the loss of water weight. While this initial weight loss may not represent true fat loss, it can still provide motivation and encouragement for individuals beginning their weight loss journey.

- **Disease Prevention**

The carnivore diet's impact on disease prevention extends beyond metabolic health and weight management to encompass various chronic diseases and health conditions:

Cardiovascular Disease: Contrary to conventional wisdom, emerging research suggests that dietary saturated fat may not be as strongly linked to heart disease as once thought. The carnivore diet's emphasis on animal foods rich in saturated fat may not necessarily increase the risk of cardiovascular disease, particularly when combined with other lifestyle factors such as regular physical activity and avoidance of smoking.

Type 2 Diabetes: By promoting weight loss, improving insulin sensitivity, and stabilizing blood glucose levels, the carnivore diet may help prevent and manage type 2 diabetes. Some studies have shown that low-carbohydrate diets can lead to significant reductions in HbA1c levels and medication requirements in individuals with diabetes.

Autoimmune Disorders: Certain autoimmune disorders, such as rheumatoid arthritis, inflammatory bowel disease, and psoriasis, involve dysregulated immune responses and chronic inflammation. The carnivore diet's elimination of potentially inflammatory plant foods may help alleviate symptoms and improve quality of life in individuals with autoimmune conditions.

Gastrointestinal Disorders: The carnivore diet's simplicity and elimination of common dietary irritants such as gluten, dairy, and fiber-rich plant foods may benefit individuals with gastrointestinal disorders such as irritable bowel syndrome (IBS), Crohn's disease, and ulcerative colitis. Some anecdotal reports suggest that symptoms such as bloating, gas, and diarrhea may improve on a carnivore diet.

The carnivore diet has the potential to positively impact metabolic health, weight management, and disease prevention through various mechanisms. By prioritizing animal foods rich in protein and healthy fats while eliminating carbohydrates and potentially inflammatory plant foods, the carnivore diet may improve insulin sensitivity, stabilize blood glucose levels, promote weight loss, preserve lean body mass, and reduce the risk of chronic diseases such as cardiovascular disease, type 2 diabetes, autoimmune disorders, and gastrointestinal disorders.

However, it's essential to recognize that the carnivore diet is not without controversy and potential drawbacks. Long-term adherence to a strict carnivore diet may lead to nutrient deficiencies, digestive issues, and other health complications, particularly if not properly planned and supervised. Additionally, individual responses to the diet can vary, and not everyone may experience the same benefits or tolerate the dietary restrictions.

Further research is needed to better understand the long-term effects and safety of the carnivore diet, as well as its role in the context of overall dietary patterns and lifestyle factors. Individuals considering the carnivore diet should consult with healthcare professionals, monitor their health closely, and make informed decisions based on their individual health needs and preferences. Ultimately, achieving optimal health and well-being requires a personalized approach that takes into account individual differences, dietary preferences, and lifestyle factors.

Comparisons with other dietary approaches (e.g., keto, paleo)

Comparing the carnivore diet with other dietary approaches such as keto and paleo provides valuable insights into their similarities, differences, and potential benefits and drawbacks. While these dietary approaches share some common principles, they also have distinct features and varying effects on health outcomes. In this section, we will explore the carnivore diet in comparison to the keto and paleo diets, examining their macronutrient compositions, food choices, metabolic effects, potential health benefits, and considerations for long-term adherence.

- **Ketogenic Diet (Keto)**

The ketogenic diet is a high-fat, moderate-protein, low-carbohydrate dietary approach designed to induce ketosis, a metabolic state characterized by the production of ketone bodies from fat breakdown. While the carnivore diet is inherently ketogenic due to its minimal carbohydrate intake, there are notable differences between the two diets:

Macronutrient Composition: Both the carnivore diet and the ketogenic diet emphasize high fat intake, but the carnivore diet typically contains lower overall carbohydrate intake, as it excludes plant-based foods altogether. The ketogenic diet typically allows for a small amount of carbohydrates, often ranging from 20 to 50 grams per day, primarily from non-starchy vegetables, nuts, and seeds.

Food Choices: While both diets prioritize animal-derived foods such as meat, fish, and eggs, the ketogenic diet allows for a broader range of food choices, including non-starchy vegetables, nuts, seeds, dairy products, and low-carbohydrate fruits such as berries. In contrast, the carnivore diet restricts food choices exclusively to animal foods, eliminating all plant-based foods and their derivatives.

Metabolic Effects: Both the carnivore diet and the ketogenic diet can induce ketosis and shift the body's primary fuel source from carbohydrates to fat. Ketosis is associated with various metabolic benefits, including improved insulin sensitivity, stabilized blood glucose levels, enhanced fat oxidation, and appetite suppression. However, the degree of ketosis and metabolic effects may differ between individuals following a carnivore diet versus a ketogenic diet due to differences in carbohydrate intake and food composition.

Health Benefits: Both the carnivore diet and the ketogenic diet have been associated with several health benefits, including weight loss, improved metabolic markers, reduced inflammation, and enhanced cognitive function. Research suggests that ketogenic diets may be effective for epilepsy management, neuroprotection, and certain metabolic conditions such as type 2 diabetes and metabolic syndrome. While the carnivore diet shares some of these potential benefits, further research is needed to elucidate its long-term effects and safety.

Considerations: Individuals considering a ketogenic diet should be mindful of their carbohydrate intake, monitor ketone levels, and ensure an adequate intake of micronutrients such as electrolytes, vitamins, and minerals. Similarly, those following a carnivore diet should pay attention to nutrient intake, particularly fiber, vitamin C, and phytonutrients found in plant-based foods. Both diets may require supplementation and careful monitoring to prevent nutrient deficiencies and optimize health outcomes.

- **Paleo Diet**

The paleo diet, also known as the "caveman" or "Stone Age" diet, aims to emulate the dietary patterns of our Paleolithic ancestors by focusing on whole, unprocessed foods that were available during the pre-agricultural era. While there are similarities between the carnivore diet and the paleo diet, there are also key differences:

Food Choices: Both the carnivore diet and the paleo diet prioritize whole, nutrient-dense foods and exclude processed and refined foods. However, the carnivore diet is more restrictive in terms of food choices, as it excludes all plant-based foods and their derivatives. In contrast, the paleo diet allows for a wider variety of foods, including fruits, vegetables, nuts, seeds, lean meats, fish, and healthy fats.

Macronutrient Composition: The paleo diet typically includes a balanced macronutrient ratio, with an emphasis on protein, healthy fats, and unprocessed carbohydrates from fruits and vegetables. In contrast, the carnivore diet is higher in protein and fat and virtually devoid of carbohydrates, aside from trace amounts found in animal foods. The macronutrient composition of the carnivore diet may vary depending on individual food choices and preferences.

Metabolic Effects: While both the carnivore diet and the paleo diet can promote weight loss and improve metabolic health, they may exert different metabolic effects due to variations in macronutrient composition and food choices. The paleo diet's inclusion of carbohydrates from fruits and vegetables may provide more dietary flexibility and support physical activity levels, whereas the carnivore diet's emphasis on protein and fat may promote greater satiety and fat loss.

Health Benefits: Both the carnivore diet and the paleo diet have been associated with several health benefits, including improved insulin sensitivity, reduced inflammation, and enhanced nutrient intake from whole foods. The paleo diet's focus on whole, unprocessed foods may help reduce the risk of chronic diseases such as obesity, type 2 diabetes, cardiovascular disease, and autoimmune disorders. While the carnivore diet shares some of these potential benefits, its exclusion of plant-based foods may raise concerns about nutrient deficiencies and long-term health effects.

Considerations: Individuals following a paleo diet should prioritize high-quality, nutrient-dense foods and emphasize variety to ensure adequate intake of essential nutrients. While the paleo diet allows for greater dietary flexibility compared to the carnivore diet, individuals should still be mindful of their carbohydrate intake and choose nutrient-rich sources of carbohydrates such as fruits and vegetables. Additionally, incorporating regular physical activity and adopting a balanced lifestyle are essential components of a healthy paleo diet.

Comparing the carnivore diet with other dietary approaches such as keto and paleo provides valuable insights into their similarities, differences, and potential implications for health and well-being. While all three dietary approaches share some common principles, such as prioritizing whole, nutrient-dense foods and excluding processed and refined foods, they also have distinct features and varying effects on metabolic health, weight management, and disease prevention.

The carnivore diet's emphasis on animal-derived foods and exclusion of plant-based foods may induce ketosis and promote weight loss, but it also raises concerns about nutrient deficiencies and long-term health effects. In contrast, the ketogenic diet and the paleo diet offer greater dietary flexibility and include a wider variety of foods, allowing for more balanced macronutrient ratios and potentially improved adherence and sustainability.

Ultimately, the choice of dietary approach should be individualized based on personal preferences, health goals, and metabolic considerations. Consulting with healthcare professionals, monitoring health markers, and making informed decisions about dietary choices are essential for optimizing health outcomes and promoting long-term well-being. Further research is needed to elucidate the effects of these dietary approaches on various health outcomes and to better understand their role in the context of overall dietary patterns and lifestyle factors.

Chapter 4

Transitioning to a Carnivore Lifestyle

Preparing mentally and emotionally for the shift

Transitioning to a carnivore diet involves more than just changing what you eat; it requires mental and emotional preparation to navigate the challenges and adjustments that come with such a significant dietary shift. In this part, we will delve into the various aspects of preparing oneself mentally and emotionally for transitioning to a carnivore diet, exploring the motivations behind this dietary choice, potential challenges, strategies for success, and the importance of self-awareness and support.

- **Understanding the Motivation**

Before embarking on any significant lifestyle change, it's crucial to understand the motivation behind it. People may choose to adopt a carnivore diet for various reasons, including health concerns, ethical beliefs, environmental considerations, or simply curiosity about its potential benefits. Whatever the reason, having a clear understanding of why one is making this change can provide the foundation for mental and emotional preparation.

- **Managing Expectations**

  Transitioning to a carnivore diet is not without its challenges, and it's essential to manage expectations from the outset. While some people may experience rapid improvements in health and well-being, others may face initial discomfort or adjustment periods as their bodies adapt to the new way of eating. Recognizing that everyone's experience will be different and that results may vary can help in maintaining realistic expectations and staying motivated during the transition.

- **Educating Oneself**

  A well-informed approach is key to success when transitioning to a carnivore diet. Educating oneself about the nutritional aspects of a meat-based diet, including the importance of sourcing high-quality animal products and ensuring adequate nutrient intake, can provide the knowledge needed to make informed choices and optimize health outcomes. Understanding the potential benefits and risks associated with a carnivore diet can also help in making decisions that align with one's individual health goals and values.

- **Overcoming Social and Cultural Challenges**

One of the most significant challenges of transitioning to a carnivore diet can be social and cultural pressure. In a society where plant-based diets are often promoted as the healthiest option and meat consumption is sometimes stigmatized, individuals may face skepticism or criticism from friends, family, and peers. It's essential to mentally prepare for these challenges and develop strategies for navigating social situations, such as politely declining non-carnivore foods and confidently explaining one's dietary choices when necessary.

- **Building a Support System**

Having a supportive network can make a significant difference when transitioning to a carnivore diet. Whether it's finding like-minded individuals online or connecting with friends and family members who are understanding and supportive of your dietary choices, having people to share experiences with, seek advice from, and lean on for support can help in staying motivated and overcoming challenges along the way.

- **Practicing Self-Care**

Transitioning to a new diet can be physically and emotionally taxing, so it's essential to prioritize self-care throughout the process. This includes getting plenty of rest, managing stress through relaxation techniques or mindfulness practices, and engaging in activities that bring joy and fulfillment. Taking care of oneself holistically can help in maintaining mental and emotional well-being during times of change and adjustment.

- **Embracing Flexibility**

While the carnivore diet is often portrayed as strict and regimented, it's essential to remember that flexibility can be key to long-term success. Rather than viewing the diet as a set of rigid rules to be followed without deviation, it can be helpful to approach it with a mindset of flexibility and adaptation. This might mean experimenting with different types of animal products, incorporating occasional deviations from strict carnivory, or adjusting the diet based on individual preferences and needs.

- **Celebrating Successes**

Transitioning to a carnivore diet is a significant achievement, and it's essential to celebrate successes along the way. Whether it's noticing improvements in energy levels, achieving weight loss goals, or experiencing other positive changes in health and well-being, taking the time to acknowledge and celebrate these accomplishments can help in staying motivated and reinforcing the commitment to the new way of eating.

Preparing mentally and emotionally for the shift to a carnivore diet involves understanding one's motivations, managing expectations, educating oneself, overcoming social and cultural challenges, building a support system, practicing self-care, embracing flexibility, and celebrating successes along the way. By approaching the transition with mindfulness, resilience, and a willingness to adapt, individuals can navigate the challenges and

reap the potential benefits of a meat-based diet

while maintaining overall well-being and

satisfaction with their dietary choices.

Chapter 5

Breakfast Recipes

Perfectly Seared Ribeye Steak with Grass-Fed Butter

Description: This recipe yields a succulent and flavorful ribeye steak with a perfectly seared crust and a rich grass-fed butter finish.

Preparation time: 10 minutes

Cooking time: 10 minutes

Ingredients:

- 2 ribeye steaks (about 1 inch thick)

- Salt and freshly ground black pepper to taste

- 2 tablespoons grass-fed butter

- Optional: minced garlic, thyme, or rosemary for additional flavor

Directions:

1. Preheat your air fryer to 400°F (200°C) for about 5 minutes.

2. Season both sides of the ribeye steaks generously with salt and pepper.

3. Place the steaks in the air fryer basket in a single layer, ensuring they're not overcrowded.

4. Cook the steaks for 4-5 minutes for medium-rare, flipping halfway through the cooking time for even searing.

5. Once the steaks reach your desired doneness, remove them from the air fryer and let them rest for a few minutes.

6. While the steaks are resting, melt the grass-fed butter in a small saucepan or microwave.

7. Drizzle the melted butter over the steaks and let it soak in for added richness.

8. Serve the ribeye steaks hot and enjoy!

Nutritional values: (per serving, approximate)

- Calories: 450

- Fat: 35g

- Protein: 35g

- Carbohydrates: 0g

- Fiber: 0g

Easy Air Fryer Carnivore Meatballs

Description: These carnivore meatballs are simple to make and bursting with flavor, making them a perfect keto-friendly snack or meal option.

Preparation time: 10 minutes

Cooking time: 15 minutes

Ingredients:

- 1 pound ground beef

- Salt and pepper to taste

- Optional: garlic powder, onion powder, or other preferred seasonings

Directions:

1. Preheat your air fryer to 375°F (190°C).

2. In a mixing bowl, combine the ground beef with salt, pepper, and any additional seasonings of your choice.

3. Form the seasoned ground beef into small meatballs, about 1 inch in diameter.

4. Place the meatballs in the air fryer basket in a single layer, ensuring they're not touching each other.

5. Cook the meatballs in the air fryer for 12-15 minutes, shaking the basket halfway through to ensure even cooking.

6. Once the meatballs are cooked through and nicely browned, remove them from the air fryer.

7. Serve hot as a snack or with your favorite carnivore-friendly sauce.

Nutritional values: (per serving, approximate)

- Calories: 250

- Fat: 20g

- Protein: 18g

- Carbohydrates: 0g

- Fiber: 0g

(Note: Nutritional values may vary depending on the specific type of ground beef used.)

Keto Carnivore Waffle

Description: This carnivore waffle recipe is low in carbs and packed with protein, making it a delicious and satisfying breakfast option for those following a keto or carnivore diet.

Preparation time: 5 minutes

Cooking time: 10 minutes

Ingredients:

- 4 large eggs

- 1/4 cup grated cheese (optional)

- Salt and pepper to taste

- Cooking spray or butter for greasing the waffle iron

Directions:

1. Preheat your waffle iron according to the manufacturer's instructions.

2. In a mixing bowl, whisk together the eggs, grated cheese (if using), salt, and pepper until well combined.

3. Lightly grease the preheated waffle iron with cooking spray or butter.

4. Pour the egg mixture evenly onto the waffle iron and close the lid.

5. Cook the waffle for about 5-7 minutes or until golden brown and cooked through.

6. Carefully remove the cooked waffle from the iron and repeat with the remaining egg mixture if needed.

7. Serve the keto carnivore waffle hot with your favorite toppings or enjoy it as is.

Nutritional values: (per serving, approximate)

- Calories: 250

- Fat: 20g

- Protein: 18g

- Carbohydrates: 1g

- Fiber: 0g

Carnivore Beef Liver Pancakes

Description: These beef liver pancakes are a creative and delicious way to incorporate nutrient-rich organ meat into your diet, perfect for those following a carnivore or keto lifestyle.

Preparation time: 15 minutes

Cooking time: 15 minutes

Ingredients:

- 1 pound beef liver, trimmed and sliced

- 2 large eggs

- Salt and pepper to taste

- Cooking fat (e.g., tallow, lard, butter) for frying

Directions:

1. In a blender or food processor, combine the beef liver slices, eggs, salt, and pepper.

2. Blend the mixture until smooth and well combined, resembling a pancake batter consistency.

3. Heat a skillet or frying pan over medium heat and add a generous amount of cooking fat to grease the surface.

4. Pour the beef liver batter onto the hot skillet, forming pancakes of your desired size.

5. Cook the pancakes for 3-4 minutes on each side or until golden brown and cooked through.

6. Once cooked, transfer the beef liver pancakes to a plate and repeat the process with any remaining batter.

7. Serve the carnivore beef liver pancakes hot with your favorite garnishes or sauces.

Nutritional values: (per serving, approximate)

- Calories: 200

- Fat: 8g

- Protein: 30g

- Carbohydrates: 2g

- Fiber: 0g

"Meat Lovers" Carnivore Pizza

Description: This carnivore pizza is a hearty and satisfying dish loaded with meaty toppings, perfect for satisfying your cravings while staying true to your carnivore diet.

Preparation time: 20 minutes

Cooking time: 15 minutes

Ingredients:

- 1 pound ground beef

- 1 pound ground pork

- Salt and pepper to taste

- 1 cup sugar-free marinara sauce

- 1 cup shredded mozzarella cheese

- Optional: sliced pepperoni, cooked bacon, cooked sausage, sliced mushrooms, or other preferred toppings

Directions:

1. Preheat your oven to 400°F (200°C).

2. In a mixing bowl, combine the ground beef and ground pork with salt and pepper, mixing until well combined.

3. Press the meat mixture onto a parchment-lined baking sheet, forming a thin crust shape.

4. Bake the meat crust in the preheated oven for 10-12 minutes or until cooked through and slightly crispy.

5. Remove the meat crust from the oven and spread the sugar-free marinara sauce evenly over the surface.

6. Sprinkle the shredded mozzarella cheese over the sauce, followed by your desired meat toppings.

7. Return the pizza to the oven and bake for an additional 5-7 minutes or until the cheese is melted and bubbly.

8. Once cooked, remove the carnivore pizza from the oven and let it cool slightly before slicing.

9. Serve hot and enjoy the meaty goodness!

Nutritional values: (per serving, approximate)

- Calories: 450

- Fat: 35g

- Protein: 30g

- Carbohydrates: 2g

- Fiber: 0g

Succulent Braised Short Ribs

Description: These succulent braised short ribs are tender, flavorful, and perfect for a cozy dinner at home.

Preparation time: 20 minutes

Cooking time: 3 hours

Ingredients:

- 4 pounds beef short ribs

- Salt and pepper to taste

- 2 tablespoons cooking fat (e.g., tallow, lard, olive oil)

- 1 onion, chopped

- 2 carrots, chopped

- 2 stalks celery, chopped

- 4 cloves garlic, minced

- 2 cups beef broth

- 1 cup red wine (optional)

- 2 sprigs fresh thyme

- 2 sprigs fresh rosemary

- 2 bay leaves

Directions:

1. Preheat your oven to 325°F (160°C).

2. Season the short ribs generously with salt and pepper.

3. Heat the cooking fat in a large oven-safe Dutch oven over medium-high heat.

4. Brown the short ribs on all sides in the Dutch oven, working in batches if necessary to avoid overcrowding.

5. Once browned, transfer the short ribs to a plate and set aside.

6. In the same Dutch oven, add the chopped onion, carrots, celery, and garlic. Cook for 5-7 minutes or until the vegetables are softened.

7. Return the short ribs to the Dutch oven and pour in the beef broth and red wine (if using),

scraping up any browned bits from the bottom
of the pot.

8. Add the fresh thyme, rosemary, and bay leaves
    to the pot, then cover with a lid.

9. Transfer the Dutch oven to the preheated oven
    and braise the short ribs for 2.5 to 3 hours or
    until the meat is fork-tender.

10. Once cooked, remove the short ribs from the
    oven and let them rest for a few minutes before
    serving.

11. Serve the succulent braised short ribs hot,
    accompanied by your favorite side dishes.
    Nutritional values: (per serving, approximate)

- Calories: 450

- Fat: 35g

- Protein: 30g

- Carbohydrates: 5g

- Fiber: 1g

Carnivore Egg Pudding

Description: This carnivore egg pudding is a creamy and satisfying dessert or snack option that's both delicious and nutritious.

Preparation time: 5 minutes

Cooking time: 30 minutes

Ingredients:

- 6 large eggs

- 1 cup heavy cream

- Salt to taste

- Optional: vanilla extract or other preferred flavorings

Directions:

1. Preheat your oven to 325°F (160°C).

2. In a mixing bowl, whisk together the eggs, heavy cream, salt, and any optional flavorings until well combined.

3. Pour the egg mixture into individual ramekins or a baking dish.

4. Place the ramekins or baking dish in a larger baking pan and fill the pan with hot water until it reaches halfway up the sides of the ramekins or dish.

5. Carefully transfer the baking pan to the preheated oven and bake the egg pudding for 25-30 minutes or until set.

6. Once cooked, remove the egg pudding from the oven and let it cool slightly before serving.

7. Serve the carnivore egg pudding warm or chilled, garnished with a sprinkle of salt if desired.

Nutritional values: (per serving, approximate)

- Calories: 250

- Fat: 20g

- Protein: 12g

- Carbohydrates: 2g

- Fiber: 0g

Classic Organ Meat Pie

Description: This classic organ meat pie is a hearty and flavorful dish that's perfect for showcasing the richness of organ meats in a comforting pie format.

Preparation time: 30 minutes

Cooking time: 1 hour 30 minutes

Ingredients:

- 1 pound beef liver, diced

- 1 pound beef heart, diced

- 1 pound beef kidney, diced

- Salt and pepper to taste

- 2 tablespoons cooking fat (e.g., tallow, lard, butter)

- 1 onion, chopped

- 2 cloves garlic, minced

- 2 carrots, diced

- 2 stalks celery, diced

- 2 cups beef broth

- 1 tablespoon tomato paste

- 1 teaspoon dried thyme

- 1 teaspoon dried rosemary

- 1 sheet prepared pie crust or homemade pie dough

Directions:

1. Preheat your oven to 375°F (190°C).

2. Season the diced beef liver, heart, and kidney with salt and pepper.

3. Heat the cooking fat in a large skillet over medium-high heat.

4. Add the seasoned organ meats to the skillet and cook until browned on all sides. Remove from the skillet and set aside.

5. In the same skillet, add the chopped onion, garlic, carrots, and celery. Cook for 5-7 minutes or until the vegetables are softened.

6. Return the cooked organ meats to the skillet and add the beef broth, tomato paste, dried thyme, and dried rosemary. Stir to combine.

7. Simmer the mixture for 10-15 minutes, allowing the flavors to meld and the liquid to reduce slightly.

8. Transfer the organ meat filling to a baking dish or pie plate.

9. Roll out the prepared pie crust or homemade pie dough and place it over the filling, crimping the edges to seal.

10. Cut a few slits in the top of the crust to allow steam to escape.

11. Bake the organ meat pie in the preheated oven for 45-60 minutes or until the crust is golden brown and the filling is bubbling.

12. Once cooked, remove the pie from the oven and let it cool for a few minutes before serving.

13. Slice and serve the classic organ meat pie hot, accompanied by your favorite side dishes.

Nutritional values: (per serving, approximate)

- Calories: 350

- Fat: 20g

- Protein: 25g

- Carbohydrates: 15g

- Fiber: 2g

Oven-Roasted Bone Marrow

Description: This oven-roasted bone marrow is a decadent and flavorful dish that's perfect as an appetizer or a special treat for any carnivore meal.

Preparation time: 10 minutes

Cooking time: 20 minutes

Ingredients:

- 4 beef marrow bones, cut lengthwise

- Salt and pepper to taste

- Optional: minced garlic, chopped parsley, lemon wedges

Directions:

1. Preheat your oven to 425°F (220°C).

2. Place the marrow bones on a baking sheet, cut side up.

3. Season the marrow generously with salt and pepper.

4. Roast the marrow bones in the preheated oven for 15-20 minutes or until the marrow is soft and starting to brown.

5. Once cooked, remove the bone marrow from the oven and let it cool for a few minutes.

6. Serve the oven-roasted bone marrow hot, accompanied by optional garnishes such as

minced garlic, chopped parsley, and lemon wedges.

7. Spread the soft marrow on toast or enjoy it straight from the bone with a spoon.

Nutritional values: (per serving, approximate)

- Calories: 250

- Fat: 20g

- Protein: 15g

- Carbohydrates: 0g

- Fiber: 0g

Grass-fed Beef Liver Chips

Description: These grass-fed beef liver chips are a crunchy and nutritious snack that's perfect for satisfying your cravings while staying true to your carnivore diet.

Preparation time: 10 minutes

Cooking time: 20 minutes

Ingredients:

- 1 pound grass-fed beef liver, thinly sliced

- Salt and pepper to taste

- Cooking fat (e.g., tallow, lard, butter) for frying

Directions:

1. Preheat your oven to 250°F (120°C).

2. Place the thinly sliced beef liver on a baking sheet lined with parchment paper.

3. Season the liver slices with salt and pepper to taste.

4. Bake the liver slices in the preheated oven for 15-20 minutes or until they are dried and crispy.

5. While the liver chips are baking, heat the cooking fat in a skillet over medium-high heat.

6. Once the liver chips are crispy, remove them from the oven and transfer them to the hot skillet.

7. Fry the liver chips in the skillet for 1-2 minutes on each side or until they are golden brown and crispy.

8. Once cooked, remove the liver chips from the skillet and drain them on a paper towel-lined plate to remove excess grease.

9. Serve the grass-fed beef liver chips hot as a crunchy snack or appetizer.

Nutritional values: (per serving, approximate)

- Calories: 200

- Fat: 10g

- Protein: 25g

- Carbohydrates: 1g

- Fiber: 0g

Carnivore Diet Breakfast Sandwich

Description: This carnivore diet breakfast sandwich is a hearty and satisfying meal option, perfect for starting your day with a protein-packed boost.

Preparation time: 10 minutes

Cooking time: 15 minutes

Ingredients:

- 2 large eggs

- 4 slices bacon

- 2 slices cheese (optional)

- Salt and pepper to taste

- Cooking fat (e.g., tallow, lard, butter) for frying

Directions:

1. Heat a skillet over medium heat and cook the bacon until crispy. Remove from the skillet and set aside.

2. In the same skillet, melt a tablespoon of cooking fat.

3. Crack the eggs into the skillet and cook them to your desired doneness, seasoning with salt and pepper.

4. Once the eggs are cooked, assemble the breakfast sandwich by placing the cooked bacon and optional cheese slices between two fried eggs.

5. Serve the carnivore diet breakfast sandwich hot and enjoy!

Nutritional values: (per serving, approximate)

- Calories: 450

- Fat: 35g

- Protein: 25g

- Carbohydrates: 1g

- Fiber: 0g

Carnivore Steak Nuggets

Description: These carnivore steak nuggets are bite-sized pieces of tender and flavorful steak, perfect for snacking or as a protein-packed addition to any meal.

Preparation time: 10 minutes

Cooking time: 10 minutes

Ingredients:

- 1 pound steak (e.g., ribeye, sirloin), cut into bite-sized pieces

- Salt and pepper to taste

- Cooking fat (e.g., tallow, lard, butter) for frying

Directions:

1. Season the steak pieces with salt and pepper to taste.

2. Heat a skillet over medium-high heat and add
    a tablespoon of cooking fat.

3. Once the skillet is hot, add the seasoned steak
    pieces in a single layer, ensuring they are not
    overcrowded.

4. Cook the steak nuggets for 2-3 minutes on
    each side or until they are browned and cooked
    to your desired level of doneness.

5. Once cooked, remove the steak nuggets from
    the skillet and let them rest for a few minutes
    before serving.

6. Serve the carnivore steak nuggets hot as a
    snack or alongside your favorite dipping sauce.
    Nutritional values: (per serving, approximate)

- Calories: 300

- Fat: 20g

- Protein: 30g

- Carbohydrates: 0g

- Fiber: 0g

Grass-Fed Beef Stroganoff

Description: This grass-fed beef stroganoff is a comforting and satisfying dish, featuring tender beef cooked in a creamy sauce, perfect for a cozy dinner at home.

Preparation time: 15 minutes

Cooking time: 30 minutes

Ingredients:

- 1 pound grass-fed beef sirloin, thinly sliced

- Salt and pepper to taste

- 2 tablespoons cooking fat (e.g., tallow, lard, butter)

- 1 onion, thinly sliced

- 2 cloves garlic, minced

- 8 ounces mushrooms, sliced

- 1 cup beef broth

- 1 cup heavy cream

- 2 tablespoons sour cream (optional)

- 2 tablespoons Dijon mustard

- Fresh parsley, chopped, for garnish

Directions:

1. Season the thinly sliced beef sirloin with salt and pepper to taste.

2. Heat a large skillet over medium-high heat and add a tablespoon of cooking fat.

3. Once the skillet is hot, add the seasoned beef slices in a single layer and cook for 2-3 minutes on each side until browned. Remove the beef from the skillet and set aside.

4. In the same skillet, add another tablespoon of cooking fat if needed and sauté the thinly sliced onion until softened.

5. Add the minced garlic and sliced mushrooms to the skillet and cook for an additional 5 minutes until the mushrooms are golden brown and tender.

6. Return the cooked beef to the skillet and pour in the beef broth, heavy cream, sour cream (if using), and Dijon mustard. Stir to combine.

7. Simmer the mixture for 10-15 minutes, allowing the flavors to meld and the sauce to thicken slightly.

8. Once cooked, remove the beef stroganoff from the heat and garnish with chopped fresh parsley.

9. Serve the grass-fed beef stroganoff hot over cauliflower rice or your preferred side dish.

Nutritional values: (per serving, approximate)

- Calories: 400

- Fat: 30g

- Protein: 25g

- Carbohydrates: 5g

- Fiber: 1g

Perfectly Grilled Lamb Chops

Description: These perfectly grilled lamb chops are tender, juicy, and bursting with flavor, making them a delicious and elegant main course for any carnivore meal.

Preparation time: 10 minutes

Cooking time: 10 minutes

Ingredients:

- 4 lamb chops

- Salt and pepper to taste

- 2 tablespoons olive oil

- Optional: minced garlic, chopped rosemary, lemon wedges for serving

Directions:

1. Preheat your grill to medium-high heat.

2. Season the lamb chops generously with salt and pepper on both sides.

3. Drizzle the olive oil over the seasoned lamb chops and rub to coat evenly.

4. Place the lamb chops on the preheated grill and cook for 4-5 minutes on each side for medium-rare or until cooked to your desired level of doneness.

5. Once cooked, remove the lamb chops from the grill and let them rest for a few minutes before serving.

6. Optional: Garnish the grilled lamb chops with minced garlic, chopped rosemary, or serve with lemon wedges for added flavor.

Nutritional values: (per serving, approximate)

- Calories: 350

- Fat: 25g

- Protein: 30g

- Carbohydrates: 0g

- Fiber: 0g

Chicken Liver Pate

Description: This chicken liver pâté is rich, creamy, and full of flavor, making it a luxurious appetizer or spread for any carnivore-friendly meal.

Preparation time: 10 minutes

Cooking time: 15 minutes

Ingredients:

- 1 pound chicken livers, trimmed

- 1/2 cup unsalted butter

- 1 onion, chopped

- 2 cloves garlic, minced

- 2 tablespoons brandy (optional)

- Salt and pepper to taste

- Fresh parsley, chopped, for garnish

Directions:

1. Rinse the chicken livers under cold water and pat them dry with paper towels.

2. In a skillet, melt 2 tablespoons of unsalted butter over medium heat.

3. Add the chopped onion and minced garlic to the skillet and cook until softened and fragrant.

4. Increase the heat to medium-high and add the chicken livers to the skillet. Cook for 5-7 minutes, stirring occasionally, until the livers are browned on the outside but still slightly pink on the inside.

5. Remove the skillet from the heat and let the mixture cool slightly.

6. Transfer the cooked chicken livers, onions, and garlic to a food processor.

7. Add the remaining unsalted butter and brandy (if using) to the food processor. Season with salt and pepper to taste.

8. Blend the mixture until smooth and creamy, scraping down the sides of the food processor as needed.

9. Once blended, transfer the chicken liver pâté to a serving dish or individual ramekins.

10. Garnish with chopped fresh parsley and cover with plastic wrap.

11. Refrigerate the pâté for at least 1-2 hours before serving to allow the flavors to meld.

12. Serve the chicken liver pâté chilled, accompanied by your favorite low-carb crackers or vegetable sticks.

Nutritional values: (per serving, approximate)

- Calories: 200

- Fat: 15g

- Protein: 15g

- Carbohydrates: 2g

- Fiber: 0g

Smokey Bacon-Wrapped Chicken Thighs

Description: These smokey bacon-wrapped chicken thighs are tender, flavorful, and easy to prepare, making them a delicious addition to any carnivore-friendly meal.

Preparation time: 10 minutes

Cooking time: 25 minutes

Ingredients:

- 4 boneless, skinless chicken thighs

- 8 slices bacon

- Salt and pepper to taste

- Smoked paprika for seasoning

Directions:

1. Preheat your oven to 400°F (200°C).

2. Season the chicken thighs with salt, pepper, and smoked paprika to taste.

3. Wrap each chicken thigh with 2 slices of bacon, ensuring the bacon completely covers the chicken.

4. Place the bacon-wrapped chicken thighs on a baking sheet lined with parchment paper.

5. Bake in the preheated oven for 20-25 minutes or until the bacon is crispy and the chicken is cooked through.

6. Once cooked, remove the bacon-wrapped chicken thighs from the oven and let them rest for a few minutes before serving.

7. Serve the smokey bacon-wrapped chicken thighs hot, accompanied by your favorite side dishes.

Nutritional values: (per serving, approximate)

- Calories: 350

- Fat: 25g

- Protein: 30g

- Carbohydrates: 0g

- Fiber: 0g

Hidden Liver Meat Muffins

Description: These hidden liver meat muffins are a sneaky way to incorporate nutrient-rich organ meat into your diet, perfect for those who want to reap the benefits of liver without the taste.

Preparation time: 15 minutes

Cooking time: 25 minutes

Ingredients:

- 1 pound ground beef

- 1/2 pound beef liver, finely chopped or ground

- 1 onion, finely chopped

- 2 cloves garlic, minced

- Salt and pepper to taste

- Cooking fat (e.g., tallow, lard, butter) for greasing

- Optional: grated cheese for topping

Directions:

1. Preheat your oven to 375°F (190°C). Grease a muffin tin with cooking fat.

2. In a mixing bowl, combine the ground beef, chopped liver, onion, garlic, salt, and pepper until well combined.

3. Divide the meat mixture evenly among the muffin cups, pressing it down to form muffin shapes.

4. Optional: Top each meat muffin with grated cheese for added flavor.

5. Bake in the preheated oven for 20-25 minutes or until the meat is cooked through and the tops are golden brown.

6. Once cooked, remove the meat muffins from the oven and let them cool for a few minutes before serving.

7. Serve the hidden liver meat muffins hot as a nutritious snack or meal option.

Nutritional values: (per serving, approximate)

- Calories: 250

- Fat: 15g

- Protein: 20g

- Carbohydrates: 2g

- Fiber: 0g

Savory Brisket Queso

Description: This savory brisket queso is a flavorful and indulgent dip, combining tender brisket with creamy cheese for a delicious carnivore-friendly appetizer or snack.

Preparation time: 15 minutes

Cooking time: 2 hours

Ingredients:

- 1 pound beef brisket, cooked and shredded

- 1 tablespoon cooking fat (e.g., tallow, lard, butter)

- 1 onion, diced

- 2 cloves garlic, minced

- 1 can (10 ounces) diced tomatoes with green chilies, drained

- 2 cups shredded cheddar cheese

- 1 cup heavy cream

- Salt and pepper to taste

- Optional: chopped fresh cilantro or green onions for garnish

Directions:

1. In a skillet, heat the cooking fat over medium heat.

2. Add the diced onion and minced garlic to the skillet and sauté until softened and fragrant.

3. Stir in the cooked and shredded brisket, allowing it to heat through.

4. Add the drained diced tomatoes with green chilies to the skillet and stir to combine.

5. Reduce the heat to low and add the shredded cheddar cheese and heavy cream to the skillet, stirring continuously until the cheese is melted and the mixture is smooth and creamy.

6. Season the brisket queso with salt and pepper to taste, adjusting as needed.

7. Once heated through and well combined, transfer the brisket queso to a serving dish.

8. Garnish with chopped fresh cilantro or green onions if desired.

9. Serve the savory brisket queso hot, accompanied by your favorite low-carb crackers or vegetable sticks.

Nutritional values: (per serving, approximate)

- Calories: 350

- Fat: 25g

- Protein: 20g

- Carbohydrates: 5g

- Fiber: 1g

Carnivore Home Cooked Mac N' Cheese

Description: This carnivore home-cooked mac n' cheese is a comforting and satisfying dish, featuring tender beef or pork cooked in a creamy cheese sauce without any noodles.

Preparation time: 10 minutes

Cooking time: 30 minutes

Ingredients:

- 1 pound ground beef or ground pork

- Salt and pepper to taste

- 2 cups shredded cheddar cheese

- 1 cup heavy cream

- 2 tablespoons butter

- Optional: chopped fresh parsley for garnish

Directions:

1. In a skillet, cook the ground beef or ground pork over medium heat until browned and cooked through. Season with salt and pepper to taste.

2. In a separate saucepan, melt the butter over medium heat.

3. Stir in the heavy cream and shredded cheddar cheese, stirring continuously until the cheese is melted and the mixture is smooth and creamy.

4. Once the cheese sauce is ready, add the cooked ground beef or pork to the saucepan, stirring to combine.

5. Continue to cook the mixture for a few minutes until heated through.

6. Once heated through and well combined, remove the carnivore mac n' cheese from the heat.

7. Garnish with chopped fresh parsley if desired.

8. Serve the carnivore home-cooked mac n' cheese hot, enjoying the creamy and cheesy goodness without any noodles.

Nutritional values: (per serving, approximate)

- Calories: 400

- Fat: 30g

- Protein: 25g

- Carbohydrates: 3g

- Fiber: 0g

Carnivore Scotch Egg

Description: This carnivore Scotch egg is a flavorful and protein-packed dish, featuring a seasoned sausage or ground meat coating around a perfectly cooked egg.

Preparation time: 15 minutes

Cooking time: 20 minutes

Ingredients:

- 4 large eggs, hard-boiled and peeled

- 1 pound ground pork or beef sausage

- Salt and pepper to taste

- Optional: herbs and spices for seasoning

- Cooking fat (e.g., tallow, lard, butter) for frying

Directions:

1. Preheat your oven to 400°F (200°C).

2. Season the ground pork or beef sausage with salt, pepper, and any desired herbs and spices. Mix well.

3. Take a portion of the seasoned sausage mixture and flatten it in your hand.

4. Encase a hard-boiled egg in the sausage mixture, ensuring an even coating.

5. Repeat for each egg, shaping them into neat rounds.

6. In a skillet, heat the cooking fat over medium-high heat.

7. Brown the sausage-coated eggs on all sides in the skillet for 2-3 minutes.

8. Transfer the browned Scotch eggs to a baking sheet and bake in the preheated oven for 15-20 minutes or until the sausage is cooked through.

9. Once cooked, remove the Scotch eggs from the oven and let them cool for a few minutes before serving.

10. Serve the carnivore Scotch eggs hot or at room temperature, sliced in half to reveal the perfectly cooked egg inside.

Nutritional values: (per serving, approximate)

- Calories: 350

- Fat: 25g

- Protein: 20g

- Carbohydrates: 0g

- Fiber: 0g

Chapter 6

Lunch Recipes

Seared Steak Salad with Chimichurri Dressing

Description: This hearty salad combines tender seared steak with vibrant chimichurri dressing, creating a flavorful and satisfying meal.

Preparation time: 15 minutes

Cooking time: 10 minutes

Ingredients:

- 1 lb flank steak

- Salt and pepper to taste

- 6 cups mixed salad greens

- 1 cup cherry tomatoes, halved

- 1/2 red onion, thinly sliced

- 1/4 cup chimichurri sauce (store-bought or homemade)

- Olive oil for cooking

Directions:

1. Season the flank steak generously with salt and pepper on both sides.

2. Heat a skillet over medium-high heat and drizzle with olive oil.

3. Once the skillet is hot, add the steak and sear for 3-4 minutes on each side for medium-rare, or adjust cooking time to your desired doneness.

4. Remove the steak from the skillet and let it rest for a few minutes before slicing thinly against the grain.

5. In a large bowl, toss the mixed salad greens, cherry tomatoes, and sliced red onion.

6. Divide the salad among plates, top with sliced steak, and drizzle chimichurri sauce over the steak.

7. Serve immediately and enjoy!

Nutritional values: (per serving)

- Calories: 350

- Protein: 25g

- Carbohydrates: 8g

- Fat: 25g

- Fiber: 3g

Tuna Melt with Keto Bread (made with almond flour)

Description: This keto-friendly tuna melt features savory tuna salad piled onto almond flour bread and topped with melted cheese, creating a satisfying low-carb meal.

Preparation time: 15 minutes

Cooking time: 15 minutes

Ingredients:

- 1 can (5 oz) tuna, drained

- 2 tablespoons mayonnaise

- 1 tablespoon chopped celery

- 1 tablespoon chopped red onion

- Salt and pepper to taste

- 4 slices keto-friendly almond flour bread

- 4 slices cheddar cheese

Directions:

1. In a bowl, mix together the tuna, mayonnaise, chopped celery, chopped red onion, salt, and pepper until well combined.

2. Preheat the oven broiler.

3. Place the almond flour bread slices on a baking sheet and toast under the broiler for 2-3 minutes on each side until lightly golden.

4. Remove the bread from the oven and divide the tuna salad evenly among the slices.

5. Top each tuna salad-topped bread slice with a slice of cheddar cheese.

6. Return the baking sheet to the broiler and broil for 2-3 minutes or until the cheese is melted and bubbly.

7. Serve hot and enjoy!

    Nutritional values: (per serving)

- Calories: 350

- Protein: 25g

- Carbohydrates: 6g

- Fat: 25g

- Fiber: 3g

Chicken Piccata with Lemon Caper Sauce

Description: This classic chicken piccata dish features tender chicken breasts cooked in a tangy lemon caper sauce, perfect for a quick and elegant dinner.

Preparation time: 10 minutes

Cooking time: 20 minutes

Ingredients:

- 4 boneless, skinless chicken breasts

- Salt and pepper to taste

- 1/2 cup all-purpose flour

- 2 tablespoons olive oil

- 4 tablespoons unsalted butter

- 1/2 cup chicken broth

- 1/4 cup fresh lemon juice

- 1/4 cup capers, drained

- 2 tablespoons chopped fresh parsley

Directions:

1. Season the chicken breasts with salt and pepper on both sides.

2. Dredge the chicken breasts in flour, shaking off any excess.

3. Heat the olive oil and 2 tablespoons of butter in a large skillet over medium-high heat.

4. Once the skillet is hot, add the chicken breasts and cook for 3-4 minutes on each side until golden brown and cooked through. Remove from the skillet and set aside.

5. In the same skillet, add the chicken broth, lemon juice, and capers, scraping up any browned bits from the bottom of the pan.

6. Simmer the sauce for 2-3 minutes until slightly reduced.

7. Return the chicken breasts to the skillet, spooning the sauce over them, and simmer for another 2-3 minutes.

8. Remove from heat, sprinkle with chopped parsley, and serve hot.

Nutritional values: (per serving)

- Calories: 350

- Protein: 25g

- Carbohydrates: 6g

- Fat: 25g

- Fiber: 3g

Beef and Shrimp Skewers with Herb Butter

Description: These flavorful skewers combine juicy beef and succulent shrimp, grilled to perfection and served with a luscious herb butter for a delicious surf and turf experience.

Preparation time: 20 minutes

Cooking time: 10 minutes

Ingredients:

- 1 lb beef sirloin, cut into 1-inch cubes

- 1 lb large shrimp, peeled and deveined

- Salt and pepper to taste

- Wooden skewers, soaked in water for 30 minutes

- 1/4 cup unsalted butter, melted

- 2 cloves garlic, minced

- 2 tablespoons chopped fresh parsley

- 1 tablespoon chopped fresh chives

Directions:

1. Preheat the grill to medium-high heat.

2. Season the beef sirloin cubes and shrimp with salt and pepper.

3. Thread the beef cubes and shrimp onto the soaked wooden skewers, alternating between beef and shrimp.

4. In a small bowl, mix together the melted butter, minced garlic, chopped parsley, and chopped chives to make the herb butter.

5. Grill the skewers for 3-4 minutes on each side, brushing with the herb butter mixture halfway through cooking, until the beef is cooked to your desired doneness and the shrimp are pink and opaque.

6. Remove the skewers from the grill and let them rest for a few minutes before serving.

7. Serve hot with any remaining herb butter on the side.

Nutritional values: (per serving)

- Calories: 350

- Protein: 25g

- Carbohydrates: 6g

- Fat: 25g

- Fiber: 3g

Grilled Lamb Burgers with Tzatziki

Description: These juicy grilled lamb burgers are seasoned to perfection and topped with creamy tzatziki sauce, making for a flavorful and satisfying meal.

Preparation time: 15 minutes

Cooking time: 10 minutes

Ingredients:

- 1 lb ground lamb

- 1/4 cup finely chopped red onion

- 2 cloves garlic, minced

- 1 tablespoon chopped fresh mint

- 1 teaspoon ground cumin

- 1/2 teaspoon ground coriander

- Salt and pepper to taste

- 4 burger buns

- Tzatziki sauce (store-bought or homemade)

- Lettuce leaves, tomato slices, and red onion slices for serving

Directions:

1. Preheat the grill to medium-high heat.

2. In a bowl, combine the ground lamb, chopped red onion, minced garlic, chopped mint, ground cumin, ground coriander, salt, and pepper. Mix until well combined.

3. Divide the lamb mixture into 4 equal portions and shape each portion into a burger patty.

4. Grill the lamb burgers for 4-5 minutes on each side, or until cooked to your desired level of doneness.

5. During the last minute of cooking, toast the burger buns on the grill until lightly golden.

6. Remove the lamb burgers and burger buns from the grill.

7. Assemble the burgers by placing a lamb patty on each bun, topping with tzatziki sauce, lettuce leaves, tomato slices, and red onion slices.

8. Serve hot and enjoy!

Nutritional values: (per serving)

- Calories: 450

- Protein: 25g

- Carbohydrates: 25g

- Fat: 25g

- Fiber: 3g

Salmon Niçoise Salad with Avocado

Description: This refreshing salad features seared salmon, tender vegetables, and creamy avocado, all drizzled with a tangy vinaigrette for a delightful Niçoise-inspired meal.

Preparation time: 20 minutes

Cooking time: 10 minutes

Ingredients:

- 1 lb salmon fillets

- Salt and pepper to taste

- 6 cups mixed salad greens

- 4 hard-boiled eggs, halved

- 1 cup cherry tomatoes, halved

- 1/2 cup Niçoise olives

- 1/4 cup thinly sliced red onion

- 1 avocado, sliced

- 1/4 cup extra virgin olive oil

- 2 tablespoons red wine vinegar

- 1 teaspoon Dijon mustard

- 1 tablespoon chopped fresh parsley

Directions:

1. Season the salmon fillets with salt and pepper on both sides.

2. Heat a skillet over medium-high heat and drizzle with olive oil.

3. Once the skillet is hot, add the salmon fillets and sear for 3-4 minutes on each side until cooked through.

4. Remove the salmon from the skillet and let it rest for a few minutes before flaking into large chunks.

5. In a large bowl, toss together the mixed salad greens, halved hard-boiled eggs, cherry tomatoes, Niçoise olives, sliced red onion, and avocado slices.

6. In a small bowl, whisk together the extra virgin olive oil, red wine vinegar, Dijon mustard, salt, and pepper to make the vinaigrette.

7. Drizzle the vinaigrette over the salad and gently toss to coat.

8. Divide the salad among plates, top with flaked salmon, sprinkle with chopped parsley, and serve immediately.

Nutritional values: (per serving)

- Calories: 400

- Protein: 25g

- Carbohydrates: 10g

- Fat: 30g

- Fiber: 6g

Chicken Fajitas with Keto Tortillas (made with almond flour)

Description: These flavorful chicken fajitas are served with keto-friendly almond flour tortillas, allowing you to enjoy a delicious Tex-Mex meal without the carbs.

Preparation time: 15 minutes

Cooking time: 15 minutes

Ingredients:

- 1 lb chicken breasts, sliced

- Salt and pepper to taste

- 2 tablespoons olive oil

- 1 bell pepper, sliced

- 1 onion, sliced

- 2 cloves garlic, minced

- 1 tablespoon chili powder

- 1 teaspoon ground cumin

- 1/2 teaspoon paprika

- 1/4 teaspoon cayenne pepper (optional)

- Keto tortillas (store-bought or homemade)

Directions:

1. Season the sliced chicken breasts with salt and pepper.

2. Heat olive oil in a large skillet over medium-high heat.

3. Add the sliced chicken breasts to the skillet and cook for 5-6 minutes until browned and cooked through. Remove from skillet and set aside.

4. In the same skillet, add the sliced bell pepper and onion. Cook for 3-4 minutes until softened.

5. Add minced garlic, chili powder, ground cumin, paprika, and cayenne pepper (if using) to the skillet. Cook for an additional minute until fragrant.

6. Return the cooked chicken to the skillet and toss to combine with the vegetables and spices.

7. Warm the keto tortillas according to package instructions or recipe.

8. Serve the chicken fajita mixture with warm keto tortillas and optional toppings such as shredded cheese, avocado slices, sour cream, and salsa.

Nutritional values: (per serving, without tortilla)

- Calories: 250

- Protein: 25g

- Carbohydrates: 5g

- Fat: 15g

- Fiber: 2g

Beef Liver Pâté on Sliced Cucumber

Description: This elegant appetizer features creamy beef liver pâté served on crisp cucumber slices for a low-carb twist on a classic favorite.

Preparation time: 15 minutes

Cooking time: 15 minutes

Ingredients:

- 1/2 lb beef liver, trimmed

- 1/4 cup unsalted butter

- 1 small onion, chopped

- 2 cloves garlic, minced

- 2 tablespoons brandy or cognac (optional)

- Salt and pepper to taste

- 1 English cucumber, sliced into rounds

- Fresh parsley for garnish

Directions:

1. Rinse the beef liver under cold water and pat dry with paper towels. Cut the liver into small pieces.

2. Heat 2 tablespoons of butter in a skillet over medium heat. Add the chopped onion and minced garlic and cook until softened, about 3-4 minutes.

3. Increase the heat to medium-high and add the beef liver to the skillet. Cook for 3-4 minutes on each side until browned but still pink in the center.

4. Remove the skillet from heat and let the liver mixture cool slightly.

5. Transfer the liver mixture to a food processor and add the remaining butter, brandy or cognac (if using), salt, and pepper. Process until smooth and creamy.

6. Refrigerate the beef liver pâté for at least 1 hour to allow flavors to meld.

7. To serve, spoon the chilled pâté onto cucumber slices and garnish with fresh parsley. Nutritional values: (per serving)

- Calories: 150

- Protein: 8g

- Carbohydrates: 4g

- Fat: 10g

- Fiber: 1g

Stuffed Peppers with Ground Beef and Cheese

Description: These flavorful stuffed peppers are filled with seasoned ground beef and topped with melted cheese for a comforting and satisfying meal.

Preparation time: 20 minutes

Cooking time: 40 minutes

Ingredients:

- 4 bell peppers, halved and seeds removed

- 1 lb ground beef

- 1 small onion, diced

- 2 cloves garlic, minced

- 1 cup cooked rice or cauliflower rice for keto version

- 1 cup tomato sauce

- 1 teaspoon Italian seasoning

- Salt and pepper to taste

- 1 cup shredded cheddar cheese

- Fresh parsley for garnish

Directions:

1. Preheat the oven to 375°F (190°C).

2. In a large skillet, cook the ground beef over medium heat until browned. Drain excess fat if necessary.

3. Add diced onion and minced garlic to the skillet with the ground beef and cook until softened, about 3-4 minutes.

4. Stir in cooked rice or cauliflower rice, tomato sauce, Italian seasoning, salt, and pepper. Cook for an additional 2-3 minutes until heated through.

5. Arrange the bell pepper halves in a baking dish, cut side up.

6. Spoon the beef mixture evenly into each bell pepper half.

7. Cover the baking dish with aluminum foil and bake in the preheated oven for 25-30 minutes until the peppers are tender.

8. Remove the foil, sprinkle shredded cheddar cheese over the stuffed peppers, and return to the oven for an additional 5-10 minutes until the cheese is melted and bubbly.

9. Garnish with fresh parsley before serving.

Nutritional values: (per serving)

- Calories: 350

- Protein: 20g

- Carbohydrates: 15g (or 5g for keto version)

- Fat: 20g

- Fiber: 3g

Creamy Chicken Soup with Bone Broth

Description: This comforting chicken soup features tender chicken, hearty vegetables, and rich bone broth, all simmered together to create a creamy and nourishing meal.

Preparation time: 15 minutes

Cooking time: 30 minutes

Ingredients:

- 1 lb boneless, skinless chicken breasts, cut into bite-sized pieces

- Salt and pepper to taste

- 2 tablespoons olive oil

- 1 onion, chopped

- 2 carrots, diced

- 2 celery stalks, diced

- 2 cloves garlic, minced

- 6 cups chicken bone broth

- 1 cup heavy cream

- 1 teaspoon dried thyme

- 1/2 teaspoon dried rosemary

- 1/2 teaspoon dried oregano

- 1/2 teaspoon dried basil

- Salt and pepper to taste

- Fresh parsley for garnish

Directions:

1. Season the chicken pieces with salt and pepper.

2. Heat olive oil in a large pot over medium heat. Add the chopped onion, diced carrots, and diced celery. Cook for 5-6 minutes until softened.

3. Add minced garlic to the pot and cook for an additional minute until fragrant.

4. Add the chicken pieces to the pot and cook until browned on all sides, about 5 minutes.

5. Pour in the chicken bone broth and bring to a simmer. Cook for 15-20 minutes until the chicken is cooked through and the vegetables are tender.

6. Stir in the heavy cream, dried thyme, dried rosemary, dried oregano, and dried basil. Season with salt and pepper to taste.

7. Simmer the soup for an additional 5 minutes to allow flavors to meld.

8. Ladle the creamy chicken soup into bowls and garnish with fresh parsley before serving.

Nutritional values: (per serving)

- Calories: 400

- Protein: 25g

- Carbohydrates: 10g

- Fat: 30g

- Fiber: 2g

Beef Empanadas with Chimichurri Sauce (without dough)

Description: These flavorful beef empanadas are made without traditional dough, instead using a seasoned ground beef filling that's packed with spices and herbs, served with a zesty chimichurri sauce.

Preparation time: 20 minutes

Cooking time: 20 minutes

Ingredients:

- 1 lb ground beef

- 1 tablespoon olive oil

- 1 onion, finely chopped

- 2 cloves garlic, minced

- 1 teaspoon ground cumin

- 1 teaspoon paprika

- 1/2 teaspoon chili powder

- Salt and pepper to taste

- 1/4 cup chopped fresh parsley

- Chimichurri sauce (store-bought or homemade)

Directions:

1. Heat olive oil in a large skillet over medium heat. Add chopped onion and minced garlic, sauté until softened.

2. Add ground beef to the skillet and cook until browned, breaking it up with a spoon as it cooks.

3. Stir in ground cumin, paprika, chili powder, salt, and pepper. Cook for another 2-3 minutes until fragrant.

4. Remove the skillet from heat and stir in chopped fresh parsley.

5. Serve the seasoned ground beef filling with chimichurri sauce for dipping.

Nutritional values: (per serving)

- Calories: 300

- Protein: 25g

- Carbohydrates: 5g

- Fat: 20g

- Fiber: 1g

Chicken Caesar Salad with Keto Croutons (made with parmesan cheese)

Description: This classic chicken Caesar salad is topped with crunchy keto-friendly parmesan cheese croutons, providing a satisfying low-carb twist on a beloved favorite.

Preparation time: 15 minutes

Cooking time: 10 minutes

Ingredients:

- 1 lb chicken breasts, grilled and sliced
- 6 cups romaine lettuce, chopped
- 1/2 cup grated parmesan cheese
- Keto Caesar dressing (store-bought or homemade)

- Keto croutons:

- 1 cup grated parmesan cheese

Directions:

1. Preheat the oven to 400°F (200°C). Line a baking sheet with parchment paper.

2. Spread grated parmesan cheese in an even layer on the prepared baking sheet.

3. Bake the parmesan cheese for 8-10 minutes until golden and crispy. Let it cool completely before breaking into crouton-sized pieces.

4. In a large bowl, toss together chopped romaine lettuce, grilled and sliced chicken breasts, and grated parmesan cheese croutons.

5. Drizzle Caesar dressing over the salad and toss to coat evenly.

6. Serve immediately and enjoy!

Nutritional values: (per serving)

- Calories: 350

- Protein: 30g

- Carbohydrates: 5g

- Fat: 20g

- Fiber: 2g

Tuna and Egg Salad Stuffed Avocados

Description: These creamy avocado halves are filled with a refreshing mixture of tuna and egg salad, creating a satisfying and nutritious low-carb meal.

Preparation time: 15 minutes

Cooking time: 10 minutes

Ingredients:

- 2 avocados, halved and pitted
- 1 can (5 oz) tuna, drained
- 2 hard-boiled eggs, chopped
- 2 tablespoons mayonnaise
- 1 tablespoon chopped fresh dill (optional)
- Salt and pepper to taste
- Lemon wedges for serving

Directions:

1. In a bowl, combine drained tuna, chopped hard-boiled eggs, mayonnaise, chopped fresh dill (if using), salt, and pepper. Mix well to combine.

2. Spoon the tuna and egg salad mixture into the avocado halves.

3. Serve stuffed avocados with lemon wedges on the side for squeezing over the top.

Nutritional values: (per serving)

- Calories: 300

- Protein: 15g

- Carbohydrates: 10g

- Fat: 25g

- Fiber: 7g

Keto Chili with Ground Beef and Sausage

Description: This hearty keto chili features a flavorful blend of ground beef and sausage, simmered with tomatoes and spices for a satisfying and comforting meal.

Preparation time: 20 minutes

Cooking time: 40 minutes

Ingredients:

- 1 lb ground beef

- 1/2 lb ground sausage

- 1 onion, chopped

- 2 cloves garlic, minced

- 1 bell pepper, chopped

- 1 can (14 oz) diced tomatoes

- 1 can (8 oz) tomato sauce

- 2 tablespoons tomato paste

- 2 teaspoons chili powder

- 1 teaspoon ground cumin

- 1/2 teaspoon paprika

- Salt and pepper to taste

- Optional toppings: shredded cheddar cheese, sour cream, chopped green onions

Directions:

1. In a large pot or Dutch oven, brown ground beef and ground sausage over medium heat, breaking it up with a spoon as it cooks.

2. Add chopped onion, minced garlic, and chopped bell pepper to the pot. Cook until vegetables are softened, about 5 minutes.

3. Stir in diced tomatoes, tomato sauce, tomato paste, chili powder, ground cumin, paprika, salt, and pepper.

4. Bring the chili to a simmer and let it cook for 30-40 minutes, stirring occasionally, until

flavors are well blended and chili has thickened.

5. Serve keto chili hot, garnished with shredded cheddar cheese, sour cream, and chopped green onions if desired.

Nutritional values: (per serving)

- Calories: 350

- Protein: 25g

- Carbohydrates: 8g

- Fat: 25g

- Fiber: 3g

Smoked Salmon Platter with Cream Cheese and Capers

Description: This elegant smoked salmon platter features thinly sliced smoked salmon served with creamy cream cheese and briny capers, perfect for a light and refreshing appetizer or brunch.

Preparation time: 10 minutes

Ingredients:

- 8 oz smoked salmon, thinly sliced

- 4 oz cream cheese

- 2 tablespoons capers

- Lemon wedges for serving

- Assorted crackers or cucumber slices for serving

Directions:

1. Arrange thinly sliced smoked salmon on a serving platter.

2. Place cream cheese in a bowl and serve alongside the smoked salmon.

3. Scatter capers over the smoked salmon.

4. Serve smoked salmon platter with lemon wedges and assorted crackers or cucumber slices.

Nutritional values: (per serving)

- Calories: 200

- Protein: 15g

- Carbohydrates: 2g

- Fat: 15g

- Fiber: 0g

Grass-Fed Beef Stew with Vegetables

Description: This hearty beef stew is made with tender grass-fed beef and a medley of flavorful vegetables, simmered together in a rich broth until everything is tender and delicious.

Preparation time: 20 minutes

Cooking time: 2 hours

Ingredients:

- 2 lbs grass-fed beef stew meat, cut into bite-sized pieces

- Salt and pepper to taste

- 2 tablespoons olive oil

- 1 onion, chopped

- 2 cloves garlic, minced

- 4 carrots, peeled and chopped

- 2 stalks celery, chopped

- 2 potatoes, peeled and diced

- 1 cup frozen peas

- 4 cups beef broth

- 2 tablespoons tomato paste

- 1 teaspoon dried thyme

- 1 teaspoon dried rosemary

- 1 bay leaf

- Chopped fresh parsley for garnish

Directions:

1. Season the beef stew meat with salt and pepper.

2. Heat olive oil in a large pot or Dutch oven over medium-high heat. Add the seasoned beef stew

meat and brown on all sides, working in
batches if necessary. Remove from pot and set
aside.

3. In the same pot, add chopped onion and
   minced garlic. Cook until softened, about 3-4
   minutes.

4. Add chopped carrots, celery, and diced
   potatoes to the pot. Cook for another 5
   minutes, stirring occasionally.

5. Return the browned beef stew meat to the pot.
   Pour in beef broth and add tomato paste, dried
   thyme, dried rosemary, and bay leaf. Stir to
   combine.

6. Bring the stew to a simmer, then reduce heat
   to low. Cover and let simmer for 1.5 to 2 hours,

stirring occasionally, until the beef is tender and the vegetables are cooked through.

7. During the last 10 minutes of cooking, add frozen peas to the pot and stir to heat through.

8. Remove the bay leaf before serving. Garnish with chopped fresh parsley and serve hot.

Nutritional values: (per serving)

- Calories: 400

- Protein: 25g

- Carbohydrates: 20g

- Fat: 20g

- Fiber: 5g

Chicken Alfredo with Broccoli and Keto Noodles (made with zucchini)

Description: This creamy chicken Alfredo dish is paired with tender broccoli and keto-friendly zucchini noodles, offering a satisfying low-carb twist on a classic favorite.

Preparation time: 15 minutes

Cooking time: 15 minutes

Ingredients:

- 1 lb chicken breasts, sliced

- Salt and pepper to taste

- 2 tablespoons olive oil

- 3 cloves garlic, minced

- 1 cup heavy cream

- 1/2 cup grated Parmesan cheese

- 2 cups broccoli florets

- 4 medium zucchinis, spiralized into noodles

- Chopped fresh parsley for garnish

Directions:

1. Season the sliced chicken breasts with salt and pepper.

2. Heat olive oil in a large skillet over medium-high heat. Add seasoned chicken slices and cook until browned and cooked through, about 5-6 minutes per side. Remove chicken from skillet and set aside.

3. In the same skillet, add minced garlic and cook until fragrant, about 1 minute.

4. Pour in heavy cream and bring to a simmer. Reduce heat to low and stir in grated Parmesan cheese until melted and smooth.

5. Add broccoli florets to the skillet and cook until tender, about 3-4 minutes.

6. Return cooked chicken slices to the skillet. Add spiralized zucchini noodles and toss to coat in the creamy Alfredo sauce. Cook for an additional 2-3 minutes until zucchini noodles are heated through.

7. Garnish with chopped fresh parsley before serving.

Nutritional values: (per serving)

- Calories: 400

- Protein: 30g

- Carbohydrates: 10g

- Fat: 25g

- Fiber: 3g

Spicy Steak Stir-Fry with Bell Peppers and Broccoli

Description: This spicy steak stir-fry features tender slices of beef cooked with vibrant bell peppers and crisp broccoli, all tossed in a zesty sauce for a flavorful and satisfying meal.

Preparation time: 20 minutes

Cooking time: 15 minutes

Ingredients:

- 1 lb flank steak, thinly sliced against the grain

- Salt and pepper to taste

- 2 tablespoons soy sauce

- 1 tablespoon sriracha sauce

- 1 tablespoon olive oil

- 1 onion, sliced

- 2 bell peppers, sliced

- 2 cups broccoli florets

- 3 cloves garlic, minced

- 1 teaspoon grated ginger

- Chopped green onions for garnish

- Sesame seeds for garnish

Directions:

1. Season the thinly sliced flank steak with salt and pepper. In a bowl, mix together soy sauce and sriracha sauce. Add the sliced steak to the sauce and toss to coat. Let it marinate for 10-15 minutes.

2. Heat olive oil in a large skillet or wok over high heat. Add marinated steak slices and cook for 2-3 minutes until browned. Remove steak from skillet and set aside.

3. In the same skillet, add sliced onion, bell peppers, and broccoli florets. Cook for 3-4 minutes until vegetables are crisp-tender.

4. Add minced garlic and grated ginger to the skillet. Cook for another minute until fragrant.

5. Return cooked steak slices to the skillet and toss everything together until heated through.

6. Garnish spicy steak stir-fry with chopped green onions and sesame seeds before serving.

Nutritional values: (per serving)

- Calories: 350

- Protein: 25g

- Carbohydrates: 15g

- Fat: 20g

- Fiber: 5g

Chicken Curry with Coconut Milk and Cauliflower Rice

Description: This flavorful chicken curry is made with tender chicken pieces simmered in a fragrant coconut milk-based sauce, served over low-carb cauliflower rice for a delicious and satisfying meal.

Preparation time: 20 minutes

Cooking time: 30 minutes

Ingredients:

- 1 lb chicken thighs, boneless and skinless, cut into bite-sized pieces

- Salt and pepper to taste

- 2 tablespoons olive oil

- 1 onion, chopped

- 3 cloves garlic, minced

- 1 tablespoon grated ginger

- 2 tablespoons curry powder

- 1 can (14 oz) coconut milk

- 1 cup chicken broth

- 2 cups cauliflower rice

- Chopped fresh cilantro for garnish

Directions:

1. Season the chicken thigh pieces with salt and pepper.

2. Heat olive oil in a large skillet over medium heat. Add chopped onion and cook until softened, about 3-4 minutes.

3. Add minced garlic and grated ginger to the skillet. Cook for another minute until fragrant.

4. Stir in curry powder and cook for 1-2 minutes until toasted and aromatic.

5. Add chicken thigh pieces to the skillet and cook until browned on all sides.

6. Pour in coconut milk and chicken broth. Bring to a simmer and let it cook for 20-25 minutes until chicken is cooked through and sauce has thickened.

7. While the curry is simmering, heat cauliflower rice in a separate skillet over medium heat until heated through.

8. Serve chicken curry over cauliflower rice, garnished with chopped fresh cilantro.

Nutritional values: (per serving)

- Calories: 400

- Protein: 20g

- Carbohydrates: 10g

- Fat: 30g

- Fiber: 5g

Grilled Fish Tacos with Cabbage Slaw and Avocado Crema

Description: These grilled fish tacos feature flaky fish fillets topped with crunchy cabbage slaw and creamy avocado crema, all wrapped in warm tortillas for a fresh and flavorful meal.

Preparation time: 20 minutes

Cooking time: 10 minutes

Ingredients:

- 1 lb white fish fillets (such as tilapia or cod)

- Salt and pepper to taste

- 2 tablespoons olive oil

- 1 teaspoon chili powder

- 1 teaspoon ground cumin

- 1/2 teaspoon paprika

- 1/4 teaspoon cayenne pepper (optional)

- 8 small tortillas (corn or flour)

Cabbage slaw:

- 2 cups shredded cabbage

- 1/4 cup chopped fresh cilantro

- 1/4 cup diced red onion

- Juice of 1 lime

- Salt to taste

Avocado crema:

- 1 ripe avocado

- 1/4 cup sour cream or Greek yogurt

- Juice of 1 lime

- Salt and pepper to taste

Directions:

1. Season fish fillets with salt, pepper, chili powder, ground cumin, paprika, and cayenne pepper (if using). Drizzle with olive oil and rub to coat evenly.

2. Preheat grill or grill pan over medium-high heat. Grill fish fillets for 3-4 minutes per side until cooked through and flaky.

3. While the fish is grilling, prepare cabbage slaw by combining shredded cabbage, chopped cilantro, diced red onion, lime juice, and salt in a bowl. Toss to coat evenly.

4. To make avocado crema, combine ripe avocado, sour cream or Greek yogurt, lime juice, salt, and pepper in a blender or food processor. Blend until smooth and creamy.

5. Warm tortillas on the grill for 1-2 minutes per side.

6. To assemble tacos, place grilled fish fillets on warm tortillas. Top with cabbage slaw and drizzle with avocado crema.

7. Serve grilled fish tacos immediately with lime wedges on the side.

Nutritional values: (per serving, without tortilla)

- Calories: 200

- Protein: 15g

- Carbohydrates: 10g

- Fat: 10g

- Fiber: 5g

Chapter 7

Dinner Recipes

Herb-Crusted Rack of Lamb with Roasted Brussels Sprouts

Description: This elegant dish features tender rack of lamb coated in a flavorful herb crust, served alongside perfectly roasted Brussels sprouts.

Preparation time: 15 minutes

Cooking time: 30 minutes

Ingredients:

- 2 racks of lamb, trimmed

- 2 tablespoons olive oil

- 2 cloves garlic, minced

- 1 tablespoon fresh rosemary, chopped

- 1 tablespoon fresh thyme, chopped

- Salt and pepper to taste

- 1 pound Brussels sprouts, trimmed and halved

- 2 tablespoons balsamic vinegar

Directions:

1. Preheat your oven to 400°F (200°C).

2. In a small bowl, mix together olive oil, garlic, rosemary, thyme, salt, and pepper.

3. Rub the herb mixture all over the racks of lamb.

4. Place the racks of lamb on a baking sheet and roast in the preheated oven for 20-25 minutes for medium-rare, or until desired doneness.

5. While the lamb is cooking, toss the Brussels sprouts with balsamic vinegar, salt, and pepper.

6. Arrange the Brussels sprouts on a separate baking sheet and roast in the oven for 20-25 minutes, or until tender and caramelized.

7. Let the lamb rest for 5-10 minutes before slicing.

8. Serve the herb-crusted rack of lamb with the roasted Brussels sprouts.

Nutritional values: (per serving)

- Calories: 450

- Fat: 28g

- Carbohydrates: 12g

- Protein: 35g

Beef Tenderloin with Roasted Rosemary Potatoes and Asparagus

Description: Juicy beef tenderloin paired with crispy roasted rosemary potatoes and tender asparagus makes for a classic and satisfying meal.

Preparation time: 20 minutes

Cooking time: 40 minutes

Ingredients:

- 4 beef tenderloin steaks

- 1 pound baby potatoes, halved

- 1 bunch asparagus, trimmed

- 3 tablespoons olive oil

- 2 tablespoons fresh rosemary, chopped

- Salt and pepper to taste

Directions:

1. Preheat your oven to 425°F (220°C).

2. Place the halved baby potatoes on a baking sheet. Drizzle with 2 tablespoons of olive oil, sprinkle with fresh rosemary, salt, and pepper, and toss to coat.

3. Roast the potatoes in the preheated oven for 25-30 minutes, or until golden and crispy.

4. Season the beef tenderloin steaks with salt and pepper.

5. Heat 1 tablespoon of olive oil in a skillet over medium-high heat. Add the steaks and sear for 3-4 minutes on each side for medium-rare, or until desired doneness.

6. While the steaks are cooking, arrange the trimmed asparagus on a separate baking sheet. Drizzle with olive oil, season with salt and pepper, and roast in the oven for 10-12 minutes, or until tender.

7. Let the steaks rest for a few minutes before serving.

8. Serve the beef tenderloin with roasted rosemary potatoes and asparagus.

Nutritional values: (per serving)

- Calories: 550

- Fat: 30g

- Carbohydrates: 25g

- Protein: 45g

Seared Scallops with Creamy Cauliflower Mash and Kale Chips

Description: Delicate seared scallops paired with creamy cauliflower mash and crispy kale chips create a harmonious blend of flavors and textures in this gourmet dish.

Preparation time: 20 minutes

Cooking time: 30 minutes

Ingredients:

- 1 pound scallops, patted dry

- 1 head cauliflower, cut into florets

- 2 tablespoons butter

- 2 cloves garlic, minced

- 1/4 cup heavy cream

- Salt and pepper to taste

- 1 bunch kale, stems removed and torn into pieces

- 2 tablespoons olive oil

Directions:

1. Start by preparing the cauliflower mash. Steam or boil the cauliflower florets until fork-tender, then drain well.

2. In a saucepan, melt the butter over medium heat. Add the minced garlic and cook for 1-2 minutes until fragrant.

3. Add the steamed cauliflower to the saucepan and mash with a potato masher or blend with an immersion blender until smooth.

4. Stir in the heavy cream and continue to cook until heated through. Season with salt and pepper to taste. Keep warm.

5. Heat the olive oil in a skillet over medium-high heat. Add the kale pieces and cook, stirring occasionally, until crispy. Remove from the skillet and drain on paper towels.

6. In the same skillet, add a bit more olive oil if needed. Pat the scallops dry with paper towels and season with salt and pepper.

7. Sear the scallops for 2-3 minutes on each side, or until golden brown and cooked through.

8. To serve, spoon the creamy cauliflower mash onto plates, top with seared scallops, and garnish with crispy kale chips.

Nutritional values: (per serving)

- Calories: 350

- Fat: 20g

- Carbohydrates: 15g

- Protein: 25g

Chicken Cordon Bleu with Keto Breadcrumbs and Parmesan Crust

Description: This classic Chicken Cordon Bleu gets a low-carb twist with keto breadcrumbs and a crispy Parmesan crust, resulting in a deliciously satisfying dish.

Preparation time: 25 minutes

Cooking time: 35 minutes

Ingredients:

- 4 boneless, skinless chicken breasts

- 4 slices Swiss cheese

- 4 slices ham

- 1/2 cup almond flour

- 1/4 cup grated Parmesan cheese

- 1 teaspoon garlic powder

- 1 teaspoon paprika

- Salt and pepper to taste

- 2 eggs, beaten

- 2 tablespoons olive oil

Directions:

1. Preheat your oven to 375°F (190°C).

2. Place each chicken breast between two sheets
    of plastic wrap and pound to 1/4-inch
    thickness using a meat mallet or rolling pin.

3. Season the chicken breasts with salt and
    pepper. Place a slice of Swiss cheese and a slice
    of ham on each chicken breast.

4. Roll up the chicken breasts tightly, securing
    with toothpicks if needed.

5. In a shallow dish, mix together almond flour,
    grated Parmesan cheese, garlic powder,
    paprika, salt, and pepper.

6. Dip each chicken breast into the beaten eggs,
    then coat with the almond flour mixture,
    pressing to adhere.

7. Heat olive oil in an oven-safe skillet over medium-high heat. Add the chicken breasts and cook for 3-4 minutes on each side, or until golden brown.

8. Transfer the skillet to the preheated oven and bake for 20-25 minutes, or until the chicken is cooked through and the crust is crispy.

9. Remove toothpicks before serving. Nutritional values: (per serving)

- Calories: 400

- Fat: 25g

- Carbohydrates: 4g

- Protein: 40g

Grilled Ribeye Steak with Chimichurri Sauce and Grilled Vegetables

Description: Juicy ribeye steak grilled to perfection, served with vibrant chimichurri sauce and a side of charred grilled vegetables, creating a feast for the senses.

Preparation time: 15 minutes

Cooking time: 15 minutes

Ingredients:

- 2 ribeye steaks

- Salt and pepper to taste

- 1 cup fresh parsley, chopped

- 4 cloves garlic, minced

- 1/4 cup red wine vinegar

- 1/2 cup olive oil

- 1 teaspoon dried oregano

- 1/2 teaspoon red pepper flakes (optional)

- Assorted vegetables for grilling (e.g., bell peppers, zucchini, onions)

Directions:

1. Preheat your grill to high heat.

2. Season the ribeye steaks generously with salt and pepper on both sides.

3. In a small bowl, combine chopped parsley, minced garlic, red wine vinegar, olive oil, dried oregano, red pepper flakes (if using), and a pinch of salt. This is your chimichurri sauce.

4. Grill the ribeye steaks over high heat for 4-5 minutes on each side for medium-rare, or until

desired doneness is reached. Remove from the grill and let rest for a few minutes.

5. While the steaks are resting, grill the assorted vegetables until tender and slightly charred, about 8-10 minutes depending on the vegetable thickness.

6. Slice the ribeye steaks against the grain and serve with a generous drizzle of chimichurri sauce and the grilled vegetables on the side.

Nutritional values: (per serving, steak only)

- Calories: 600

- Fat: 45g

- Carbohydrates: 0g

- Protein: 50g

Note: Nutritional values for vegetables and chimichurri sauce may vary depending on the types and quantities used.

Whole Roasted Chicken with Garlic and Herbs

Description: A classic roasted chicken dish infused with the flavors of garlic and aromatic herbs, resulting in tender, juicy meat and crispy golden skin.

Preparation time: 15 minutes

Cooking time: 1 hour 30 minutes

Ingredients:

- 1 whole chicken (about 4-5 pounds)

- 4 cloves garlic, minced

- 2 tablespoons fresh rosemary, chopped

- 2 tablespoons fresh thyme, chopped

- 2 tablespoons fresh parsley, chopped

- 1 lemon, sliced

- 4 tablespoons butter, softened

- Salt and pepper to taste

Directions:

1. Preheat your oven to 375°F (190°C).

2. Rinse the chicken inside and out, then pat dry with paper towels.

3. In a small bowl, mix together minced garlic, chopped rosemary, thyme, parsley, softened butter, salt, and pepper.

4. Gently loosen the skin of the chicken and rub the herb butter mixture underneath the skin and all over the chicken.

5. Place the lemon slices inside the cavity of the chicken.

6. Tie the legs together with kitchen twine and tuck the wing tips under the body of the chicken.

7. Place the chicken in a roasting pan and roast in the preheated oven for 1 hour 30 minutes, or until the internal temperature reaches 165°F (75°C) and the skin is golden brown and crispy.

8. Remove the chicken from the oven and let it rest for 10-15 minutes before carving.

9. Serve the roasted chicken with your favorite sides.

Nutritional values: (per serving)

- Calories: 400

- Fat: 25g

- Carbohydrates: 2g

- Protein: 40g

Salmon en Papillote with Lemon and Herbs

Description: Tender salmon fillets infused with the bright flavors of lemon and herbs, cooked to perfection in parchment paper parcels for a delightful and healthy meal.

Preparation time: 15 minutes

Cooking time: 20 minutes

Ingredients:

- 4 salmon fillets

- 1 lemon, thinly sliced

- 4 sprigs fresh dill

- 4 sprigs fresh thyme

- Salt and pepper to taste

- 2 tablespoons olive oil

Directions:

1. Preheat your oven to 400°F (200°C).

2. Cut four large squares of parchment paper.

3. Place a salmon fillet on each parchment square.

4. Season the salmon fillets with salt and pepper, then top each with lemon slices, fresh dill, and fresh thyme.

5. Drizzle each salmon fillet with olive oil.

6. Fold the parchment paper over the salmon and seal the edges tightly to create parcels.

7. Place the parcels on a baking sheet and bake in the preheated oven for 20 minutes, or until the salmon is cooked through and flakes easily with a fork.

8. Carefully open the parcels and transfer the salmon to serving plates.

9. Serve immediately, garnished with additional fresh herbs if desired.

Nutritional values: (per serving)

- Calories: 300

- Fat: 18g

- Carbohydrates: 2g

- Protein: 32g

Beef Bourguignon with Keto-friendly Mashed Cauliflower

Description: A hearty and comforting beef stew, slow-cooked with red wine, mushrooms, and aromatics, served with creamy mashed cauliflower as a low-carb alternative to traditional mashed potatoes.

Preparation time: 20 minutes

Cooking time: 3 hours

Ingredients:

- 2 pounds beef stew meat, cut into cubes

- 4 slices bacon, chopped

- 1 onion, chopped

- 2 carrots, peeled and sliced

- 2 cloves garlic, minced

- 1 cup red wine

- 2 cups beef broth

- 1 tablespoon tomato paste

- 1 teaspoon dried thyme

- 1 teaspoon dried rosemary

- Salt and pepper to taste

- 8 ounces mushrooms, quartered

- 1 head cauliflower, cut into florets

- 2 tablespoons butter

- 1/4 cup heavy cream

- Chopped fresh parsley for garnish

Directions:

1. In a large Dutch oven, cook the chopped bacon over medium heat until crisp. Remove the bacon with a slotted spoon and set aside, leaving the bacon fat in the pot.

2. Add the cubed beef stew meat to the pot in batches and brown on all sides. Remove the beef from the pot and set aside.

3. Add the chopped onion and sliced carrots to the pot and cook until softened, about 5 minutes. Add the minced garlic and cook for an additional minute.

4. Return the browned beef to the pot. Stir in the red wine, beef broth, tomato paste, dried thyme, dried rosemary, salt, and pepper.

5. Bring the mixture to a simmer, then cover and cook over low heat for 2-3 hours, stirring

occasionally, until the beef is tender and the sauce has thickened.

6. In the last 30 minutes of cooking, add the quartered mushrooms to the pot and continue to simmer until tender.

7. While the beef bourguignon is cooking, prepare the mashed cauliflower. Steam or boil the cauliflower florets until very tender, then drain well.

8. In a separate saucepan, melt the butter over medium heat. Add the cooked cauliflower and heavy cream, then mash with a potato masher or blend with an immersion blender until smooth.

9. Season the mashed cauliflower with salt and pepper to taste.

10. To serve, ladle the beef bourguignon over the mashed cauliflower and garnish with chopped fresh parsley and reserved crispy bacon.

Nutritional values: (per serving)

- Calories: 400

- Fat: 20g

- Carbohydrates: 8g

- Protein: 40g

Stuffed Avocados with Shrimp and Spicy Mayo

Description: Creamy avocados stuffed with seasoned shrimp and topped with a zesty spicy mayo, creating a satisfying and flavorful appetizer or light meal.

Preparation time: 20 minutes

Cooking time: 10 minutes

Ingredients:

- 2 ripe avocados

- 1/2 pound shrimp, peeled and deveined

- 1 tablespoon olive oil

- 1 teaspoon paprika

- 1/2 teaspoon garlic powder

- Salt and pepper to taste

- 1/4 cup mayonnaise

- 1 tablespoon sriracha sauce (adjust to taste)

- 1 tablespoon lime juice

- Chopped fresh cilantro for garnish

- Lime wedges for serving

Directions:

1. Cut the avocados in half lengthwise and remove the pits. Scoop out a bit of flesh from each avocado half to create a larger cavity for stuffing, being careful not to pierce through the skin.

2. In a skillet, heat olive oil over medium heat. Season the shrimp with paprika, garlic powder, salt, and pepper, then add them to the skillet. Cook the shrimp for 2-3 minutes on each side until pink and cooked through. Remove from heat and let cool slightly.

3. In a small bowl, mix together mayonnaise, sriracha sauce, and lime juice to make the spicy mayo.

4. Chop the cooked shrimp into bite-sized pieces and mix them with half of the spicy mayo.

5. Spoon the shrimp mixture into the avocado halves, dividing evenly among them.

6. Drizzle the remaining spicy mayo over the stuffed avocados.

7. Garnish with chopped fresh cilantro and serve with lime wedges on the side.

Nutritional values: (per serving, based on 1 avocado half)

- Calories: 250

- Fat: 20g

- Carbohydrates: 8g

- Protein: 10g

Grass-Fed Beef Meatloaf with Roasted Vegetables

Description: A classic comfort food favorite, this grass-fed beef meatloaf is seasoned to perfection and served with roasted vegetables for a wholesome and satisfying meal.

Preparation time: 20 minutes

Cooking time: 1 hour

Ingredients:

- 1 pound grass-fed ground beef

- 1 onion, finely chopped

- 2 cloves garlic, minced

- 1/2 cup almond flour

- 1/4 cup grated Parmesan cheese

- 1 egg, lightly beaten

- 2 tablespoons tomato paste

- 1 tablespoon Worcestershire sauce

- 1 teaspoon dried oregano

- 1 teaspoon dried thyme

- Salt and pepper to taste

- Assorted vegetables for roasting (e.g., carrots, potatoes, onions)

Directions:

1. Preheat your oven to 375°F (190°C).

2. In a large mixing bowl, combine the ground beef, chopped onion, minced garlic, almond flour, grated Parmesan cheese, beaten egg, tomato paste, Worcestershire sauce, dried

oregano, dried thyme, salt, and pepper. Mix until well combined.

3. Transfer the meat mixture to a greased loaf pan and shape it into a loaf.

4. Bake the meatloaf in the preheated oven for 45-50 minutes, or until cooked through and golden brown on top.

5. While the meatloaf is baking, prepare the assorted vegetables for roasting. Cut the vegetables into bite-sized pieces and arrange them on a baking sheet.

6. Drizzle the vegetables with olive oil and season with salt, pepper, and any desired herbs or spices.

7. Roast the vegetables in the oven alongside the meatloaf for 30-35 minutes, or until tender and caramelized.

8. Remove the meatloaf and vegetables from the oven and let rest for a few minutes before slicing.

9. Serve the sliced meatloaf with the roasted vegetables.

Nutritional values: (per serving)

- Calories: 350

- Fat: 20g

- Carbohydrates: 10g

- Protein: 25g

Grass-Fed Beef Meatloaf with Roasted Vegetables

Description: A classic comfort food favorite, this grass-fed beef meatloaf is seasoned to perfection and served with roasted vegetables for a wholesome and satisfying meal.

Preparation time: 20 minutes

Cooking time: 1 hour

Ingredients:

- 1 pound grass-fed ground beef

- 1 onion, finely chopped

- 2 cloves garlic, minced

- 1/2 cup almond flour

- 1/4 cup grated Parmesan cheese

- 1 egg, lightly beaten

- 2 tablespoons tomato paste

- 1 tablespoon Worcestershire sauce

- 1 teaspoon dried oregano

- 1 teaspoon dried thyme

- Salt and pepper to taste

- Assorted vegetables for roasting (e.g., carrots, potatoes, onions)

Directions:

1. Preheat your oven to 375°F (190°C).

2. In a large mixing bowl, combine the ground beef, chopped onion, minced garlic, almond flour, grated Parmesan cheese, beaten egg, tomato paste, Worcestershire sauce, dried

oregano, dried thyme, salt, and pepper. Mix
until well combined.

3. Transfer the meat mixture to a greased loaf pan
    and shape it into a loaf.

4. Bake the meatloaf in the preheated oven for
    45-50 minutes, or until cooked through and
    golden brown on top.

5. While the meatloaf is baking, prepare the
    assorted vegetables for roasting. Cut the
    vegetables into bite-sized pieces and arrange
    them on a baking sheet.

6. Drizzle the vegetables with olive oil and season
    with salt, pepper, and any desired herbs or
    spices.

7. Roast the vegetables in the oven alongside the meatloaf for 30-35 minutes, or until tender and caramelized.

8. Remove the meatloaf and vegetables from the oven and let rest for a few minutes before slicing.

9. Serve the sliced meatloaf with the roasted vegetables.

Nutritional values: (per serving)

- Calories: 350

- Fat: 20g

- Carbohydrates: 10g

- Protein: 25g

Herb-Roasted Chicken with Creamy Mushroom Sauce

Description: Succulent roasted chicken infused with aromatic herbs, served with a creamy mushroom sauce for a comforting and satisfying meal.

Preparation time: 15 minutes

Cooking time: 1 hour 15 minutes

Ingredients:

- 1 whole chicken (about 4-5 pounds)

- 2 tablespoons olive oil

- 2 cloves garlic, minced

- 1 tablespoon fresh thyme, chopped

- 1 tablespoon fresh rosemary, chopped

- Salt and pepper to taste

- 8 ounces mushrooms, sliced

- 2 tablespoons butter

- 2 tablespoons all-purpose flour (or almond flour for keto)

- 1 cup chicken broth

- 1/2 cup heavy cream

- Chopped fresh parsley for garnish

Directions:

1. Preheat your oven to 375°F (190°C).

2. Rinse the chicken inside and out, then pat dry with paper towels.

3. In a small bowl, mix together olive oil, minced garlic, chopped thyme, chopped rosemary, salt, and pepper.

4. Rub the herb mixture all over the chicken, including under the skin and inside the cavity.

5. Place the chicken in a roasting pan and roast in the preheated oven for 1 hour 15 minutes, or until the internal temperature reaches 165°F (75°C) and the skin is golden brown and crispy.

6. While the chicken is roasting, prepare the creamy mushroom sauce. In a skillet, melt butter over medium heat. Add the sliced mushrooms and cook until they release their juices and become golden brown.

7. Sprinkle flour over the mushrooms and stir to combine. Cook for 1-2 minutes.

8. Gradually pour in the chicken broth while stirring continuously to prevent lumps from forming.

9. Stir in the heavy cream and simmer until the sauce thickens, about 5 minutes. Season with salt and pepper to taste.

10. Once the chicken is cooked, let it rest for 10-15 minutes before carving.

11. Serve the herb-roasted chicken with the creamy mushroom sauce, garnished with chopped fresh parsley.

Nutritional values: (per serving)

- Calories: 400

- Fat: 25g

- Carbohydrates: 5g

- Protein: 35g

Pan-Seared Duck Breast with Cherry Sauce and Sautéed Greens

Description: Tender duck breast, pan-seared to perfection, served with a sweet and tangy cherry sauce and vibrant sautéed greens for an elegant and flavorful dish.

Preparation time: 15 minutes

Cooking time: 20 minutes

Ingredients:

- 2 duck breasts

- Salt and pepper to taste

- 1 cup cherries, pitted and halved

- 1/4 cup balsamic vinegar

- 2 tablespoons honey (or keto-friendly sweetener)

- 1 tablespoon olive oil

- 4 cups mixed greens (e.g., spinach, kale, Swiss chard)

- 2 cloves garlic, minced

- 1 tablespoon butter

Directions:

1. Score the skin of the duck breasts in a crosshatch pattern, being careful not to cut into the meat. Season both sides of the duck breasts generously with salt and pepper.

2. In a small saucepan, combine the cherries, balsamic vinegar, and honey. Bring to a simmer over medium heat and cook until the cherries

soften and the sauce thickens slightly, about 10 minutes. Set aside.

3. Heat olive oil in a skillet over medium-high heat. Add the duck breasts skin-side down and cook for 6-7 minutes, or until the skin is crispy and golden brown. Flip the duck breasts and cook for an additional 3-4 minutes for medium-rare, or longer to desired doneness. Remove from heat and let rest for a few minutes before slicing.

4. While the duck is resting, heat butter in a separate skillet over medium heat. Add minced garlic and sauté until fragrant, about 1 minute.

5. Add the mixed greens to the skillet and cook, stirring occasionally, until wilted, about 3-4 minutes. Season with salt and pepper to taste.

6. To serve, slice the duck breasts and arrange them on plates. Spoon the cherry sauce over the duck and serve with sautéed greens on the side.

Nutritional values: (per serving)

- Calories: 400

- Fat: 25g

- Carbohydrates: 15g

- Protein: 30g

Flank Steak Fajitas with Keto Tortillas and Guacamole

Description: Flavorful and tender flank steak, marinated and grilled to perfection, served with low-carb tortillas and creamy guacamole for a delicious twist on classic fajitas.

Preparation time: 20 minutes

Cooking time: 15 minutes

Ingredients:

For the flank steak:

- 1 pound flank steak

- 2 tablespoons olive oil

- Juice of 1 lime

- 2 cloves garlic, minced

- 1 teaspoon chili powder

- 1 teaspoon cumin

- Salt and pepper to taste

For the keto tortillas:

- 1 cup almond flour

- 2 tablespoons coconut flour

- 2 tablespoons psyllium husk powder

- 1 teaspoon baking powder

- 1/2 teaspoon salt

- 2 tablespoons olive oil

- 1/2 cup hot water

For the guacamole:

- 2 ripe avocados

- 1/4 cup diced onion

- 1/4 cup diced tomato

- 1/4 cup chopped cilantro

- Juice of 1 lime

- Salt and pepper to taste

For serving:

- Sliced bell peppers

- Sliced onions

- Sour cream (optional)

- Shredded cheese (optional)

Directions:

1. Start by marinating the flank steak. In a bowl, whisk together olive oil, lime juice, minced garlic, chili powder, cumin, salt, and pepper. Place the flank steak in a resealable plastic bag and pour the marinade over it. Seal the bag and refrigerate for at least 1 hour, or overnight for best results.

2. While the steak is marinating, prepare the keto tortillas. In a mixing bowl, combine almond flour, coconut flour, psyllium husk powder,

baking powder, and salt. Stir in olive oil and hot water until a dough forms.

3. Divide the dough into 6 equal portions and roll each portion into a ball. Place a ball of dough between two sheets of parchment paper and roll out into a thin tortilla.

4. Heat a non-stick skillet over medium-high heat. Cook each tortilla for 1-2 minutes on each side, until lightly golden brown. Set aside and keep warm.

5. Next, prepare the guacamole. Cut the avocados in half and remove the pits. Scoop the flesh into a bowl and mash with a fork. Stir in diced onion, diced tomato, chopped cilantro, lime juice, salt, and pepper.

6. Preheat your grill or skillet over medium-high heat. Remove the flank steak from the marinade and discard the excess marinade. Grill the steak for 4-5 minutes on each side, or until cooked to your desired level of doneness. Remove from heat and let rest for a few minutes before slicing.

7. While the steak is resting, sauté the sliced bell peppers and onions in a skillet until tender.

8. Slice the flank steak thinly against the grain.

9. To assemble the fajitas, place some sliced steak, sautéed vegetables, and guacamole onto each keto tortilla. Add sour cream and shredded cheese if desired.

10. Roll up the tortillas and serve immediately.

Nutritional values: (per serving, including tortillas and guacamole)

- Calories: 450

- Fat: 35g

- Carbohydrates: 10g

- Fiber: 7g

- Protein: 25g

Braised Short Ribs with Bone Marrow Broth and Roasted Root Vegetables

Description: Tender, fall-off-the-bone short ribs, braised in a rich and flavorful bone marrow broth, served with roasted root vegetables for a hearty and satisfying meal.

Preparation time: 20 minutes

Cooking time: 3 hours 30 minutes

Ingredients:

For the short ribs:

- 4 pounds beef short ribs

- Salt and pepper to taste

- 2 tablespoons olive oil

- 1 onion, chopped

- 2 carrots, chopped

- 2 stalks celery, chopped

- 4 cloves garlic, minced

- 2 cups beef broth

- 1 cup red wine

- 2 tablespoons tomato paste

- 2 sprigs fresh thyme

- 2 sprigs fresh rosemary

- 2 bay leaves

For the bone marrow broth:

- 2 pounds beef bones (marrow bones preferably)

- 1 onion, quartered

- 2 carrots, chopped

- 2 stalks celery, chopped

- 4 cloves garlic, smashed

- 2 bay leaves

- Water, enough to cover the bones

For the roasted root vegetables:

- Assorted root vegetables (e.g., carrots, parsnips, potatoes, sweet potatoes), peeled and cut into chunks

- 2 tablespoons olive oil

- Salt and pepper to taste

- Chopped fresh parsley for garnish

Directions:

1. Preheat your oven to 350°F (175°C).

2. Season the short ribs generously with salt and pepper.

3. Heat olive oil in a large Dutch oven over medium-high heat. Brown the short ribs on all sides, working in batches if necessary. Remove the short ribs from the pot and set aside.

4. In the same pot, add the chopped onion, carrots, celery, and minced garlic. Cook until softened, about 5 minutes.

5. Return the short ribs to the pot. Add beef broth, red wine, tomato paste, thyme, rosemary, and bay leaves. Bring to a simmer.

6. Cover the Dutch oven and transfer it to the preheated oven. Braise the short ribs for 3 hours, or until the meat is tender and falling off the bone.

7. While the short ribs are braising, prepare the bone marrow broth. Place beef bones, onion, carrots, celery, garlic, and bay leaves in a large stockpot. Cover with water.

8. Bring the pot to a boil, then reduce heat and simmer for 4-6 hours, skimming off any

impurities that rise to the surface. Strain the broth through a fine-mesh sieve and discard the solids.

9. For the roasted root vegetables, toss the chopped vegetables with olive oil, salt, and pepper. Spread them out on a baking sheet and roast in the preheated oven for 30-40 minutes, or until golden and tender.

10. Once the short ribs are done braising, remove them from the pot and keep warm. Skim any excess fat from the braising liquid and strain the liquid into a saucepan. Simmer the liquid over medium heat until reduced and thickened.

11. To serve, place the short ribs on plates, spoon the reduced braising liquid over them, and

garnish with chopped fresh parsley. Serve with roasted root vegetables on the side.

Nutritional values: (per serving)

- Calories: 600

- Fat: 40g

- Carbohydrates: 10g

- Protein: 50g

Baked Salmon with Lemon Dill Sauce and Asparagus

Description: Tender and flaky salmon fillets, baked to perfection and served with a light and refreshing lemon dill sauce, accompanied by roasted asparagus for a healthy and delicious meal.

Preparation time: 15 minutes

Cooking time: 15 minutes

Ingredients:

For the baked salmon:

- 4 salmon fillets

- Salt and pepper to taste

- 2 tablespoons olive oil

- 2 tablespoons lemon juice

- 2 cloves garlic, minced

- 1 teaspoon dried dill (or 1 tablespoon fresh dill)

For the lemon dill sauce:

- 1/2 cup Greek yogurt

- 2 tablespoons mayonnaise

- 1 tablespoon lemon juice

- 1 tablespoon chopped fresh dill (or 1 teaspoon dried dill)

- Salt and pepper to taste

For the roasted asparagus:

- 1 bunch asparagus, trimmed

- 1 tablespoon olive oil

- Salt and pepper to taste

Directions:

1. Preheat your oven to 400°F (200°C).

2. Season the salmon fillets with salt and pepper on both sides.

3. In a small bowl, whisk together olive oil, lemon juice, minced garlic, and dried dill.

4. Place the salmon fillets on a baking sheet lined with parchment paper. Brush the lemon dill mixture over the salmon.

5. Bake the salmon in the preheated oven for 12-15 minutes, or until the salmon is cooked through and flakes easily with a fork.

6. While the salmon is baking, prepare the lemon dill sauce. In a small bowl, mix together Greek yogurt, mayonnaise, lemon juice, chopped fresh dill, salt, and pepper. Adjust seasoning to taste.

7. For the roasted asparagus, toss trimmed asparagus spears with olive oil, salt, and pepper on a baking sheet. Roast in the oven for 10-12 minutes, or until tender and slightly browned.

8. Once the salmon is done baking, remove it from the oven and let it rest for a few minutes.

9. Serve the baked salmon with lemon dill sauce drizzled over the top and roasted asparagus on the side.

Nutritional values: (per serving)

- Calories: 300

- Fat: 15g

- Carbohydrates: 6g

- Protein: 30g

Chicken Schnitzel with Keto Breadcrumbs and Creamy Lemon Sauce

Description: Crispy chicken schnitzel coated in keto-friendly breadcrumbs, served with a creamy lemon sauce for a delightful and comforting meal.

Preparation time: 20 minutes

Cooking time: 20 minutes

Ingredients:

For the chicken schnitzel:

- 4 chicken breasts, pounded to 1/4-inch thickness

- Salt and pepper to taste

- 1/2 cup almond flour

- 1/4 cup grated Parmesan cheese

- 2 eggs, beaten

- 2 tablespoons olive oil

For the creamy lemon sauce:

- 1/2 cup heavy cream

- 2 tablespoons butter

- 2 tablespoons lemon juice

- 1 teaspoon lemon zest

- 1 tablespoon chopped fresh parsley

- Salt and pepper to taste

Directions:

1. Season the pounded chicken breasts with salt and pepper on both sides.

2. In a shallow dish, mix together almond flour and grated Parmesan cheese.

3. Dip each chicken breast in beaten eggs, then coat with the almond flour mixture, pressing gently to adhere.

4. Heat olive oil in a large skillet over medium-high heat. Add the coated chicken breasts and cook for 3-4 minutes on each side, or until golden brown and cooked through.

5. While the chicken is cooking, prepare the creamy lemon sauce. In a small saucepan, heat heavy cream and butter over medium heat until the butter is melted and the mixture is heated through.

6. Stir in lemon juice, lemon zest, chopped parsley, salt, and pepper. Simmer for a few minutes until the sauce thickens slightly.

7. Once the chicken is done cooking, transfer it to a serving platter and drizzle with the creamy lemon sauce.

8. Garnish with additional chopped parsley if desired, and serve hot.

Nutritional values: (per serving)

- Calories: 400

- Fat: 30g

- Carbohydrates: 3g

- Protein: 30g

Keto Shepherd's Pie with Ground Beef and Cauliflower Mash

Description: A low-carb twist on the classic Shepherd's Pie, made with savory ground beef filling and topped with creamy cauliflower mash, creating a comforting and satisfying dish.

Preparation time: 20 minutes

Cooking time: 40 minutes

Ingredients:

For the filling:

1. 1 pound ground beef

2. 1 onion, chopped

3. 2 cloves garlic, minced

4. 2 carrots, diced

5. 1 cup frozen peas

6. 1 cup beef broth

7. 2 tablespoons tomato paste

8. 1 tablespoon Worcestershire sauce

9. Salt and pepper to taste

For the cauliflower mash:

- 1 head cauliflower, cut into florets

- 2 tablespoons butter

- 1/4 cup heavy cream

- Salt and pepper to taste

Directions:

1. Preheat your oven to 375°F (190°C).

2. In a skillet, cook ground beef over medium heat until browned. Drain excess fat.

3. Add chopped onion, minced garlic, and diced carrots to the skillet. Cook until vegetables are softened, about 5 minutes.

4. Stir in frozen peas, beef broth, tomato paste, Worcestershire sauce, salt, and pepper. Simmer for 5-10 minutes, until the mixture thickens slightly.

5. While the filling is simmering, steam or boil cauliflower florets until very tender. Drain well.

6. In a large mixing bowl, mash the cooked cauliflower with butter, heavy cream, salt, and pepper until smooth.

7. Transfer the beef filling to a baking dish. Spread the cauliflower mash over the top.

8. Bake in the preheated oven for 20-25 minutes, or until the top is golden brown and the filling is bubbly.

9. Let cool slightly before serving.

Nutritional values: (per serving)

- Calories: 350

- Fat: 20g

- Carbohydrates: 8g

- Protein: 25g

Surf and Turf: Grilled Steak and Lobster Tails with Garlic Butter

Description: A luxurious surf and turf dish featuring perfectly grilled steak and lobster tails, served with a decadent garlic butter sauce for an indulgent dining experience.

Preparation time: 20 minutes

Cooking time: 15 minutes

Ingredients:

- 2 beef steaks (such as filet mignon or ribeye)

- 2 lobster tails

- Salt and pepper to taste

- 4 tablespoons butter, melted

- 4 cloves garlic, minced

- 1 tablespoon chopped fresh parsley

- Lemon wedges for serving

Directions:

1. Preheat your grill to medium-high heat.

2. Season the steaks and lobster tails with salt and pepper.

3. In a small bowl, mix together melted butter, minced garlic, and chopped parsley to make the garlic butter sauce.

4. Grill the steaks for 4-5 minutes on each side for medium-rare, or until desired doneness is reached. Remove from the grill and let rest for a few minutes.

5. While the steaks are resting, place the lobster tails on the grill, shell side down. Grill for 5-6 minutes, or until the meat is opaque and cooked through.

6. Serve the grilled steak and lobster tails with the garlic butter sauce and lemon wedges on the side.

Nutritional values: (per serving)

- Calories: 600

- Fat: 40g

- Carbohydrates: 2g

- Protein: 55g

One-Pan Roasted Chicken with Sausage, Onions, and Peppers

Description: An easy and flavorful one-pan meal featuring roasted chicken, sausage, onions, and peppers, seasoned with herbs and spices for a delicious dinner option.

Preparation time: 15 minutes

Cooking time: 45 minutes

Ingredients:

- 4 chicken thighs, bone-in and skin-on

- 4 chicken drumsticks, bone-in and skin-on

- 4 Italian sausages

- 2 bell peppers, sliced

- 1 onion, sliced

- 4 cloves garlic, minced

- 2 tablespoons olive oil

- 1 teaspoon dried oregano

- 1 teaspoon dried thyme

- 1 teaspoon paprika

- Salt and pepper to taste

- Chopped fresh parsley for garnish

Directions:

1. Preheat your oven to 400°F (200°C).

2. In a large mixing bowl, toss together chicken thighs, chicken drumsticks, Italian sausages, sliced bell peppers, sliced onion, minced garlic, olive oil, dried oregano, dried thyme, paprika, salt, and pepper until well coated.

3. Transfer the seasoned ingredients to a large roasting pan or baking sheet, arranging them in a single layer.

4. Roast in the preheated oven for 40-45 minutes, or until the chicken is cooked through and the sausages are browned and crispy.

5. Remove from the oven and let rest for a few minutes before serving.

6. Garnish with chopped fresh parsley before serving.

Nutritional values: (per serving)

- Calories: 500

- Fat: 35g

- Carbohydrates: 6g

- Protein: 40g

Beef Wellington with Keto Puff Pastry (made with almond flour)

Description: A gourmet dish featuring tender beef tenderloin wrapped in a flaky keto-friendly puff pastry made with almond flour, creating an impressive and delicious centerpiece for any special occasion.

Preparation time: 30 minutes

Cooking time: 45 minutes

Ingredients:

For the beef Wellington:

- 4 beef tenderloin fillets

- Salt and pepper to taste

- 2 tablespoons olive oil

- 1 tablespoon Dijon mustard

- 8 slices prosciutto

- 2 tablespoons butter

- 8 ounces mushrooms, finely chopped

- 2 cloves garlic, minced

- 2 tablespoons chopped fresh thyme

- Keto puff pastry (store-bought or homemade with almond flour)

- 1 egg, beaten (for egg wash)

For the keto puff pastry:

- 2 cups almond flour

- 1/4 cup coconut flour

- 1/4 cup psyllium husk powder

- 1/2 teaspoon salt

- 1/2 cup cold butter, diced

- 1 egg

- 1 tablespoon apple cider vinegar

- 1/4 cup cold water

Directions:

1. Preheat your oven to 400°F (200°C).

2. Season the beef tenderloin fillets with salt and pepper.

3. Heat olive oil in a skillet over high heat. Sear the fillets for 1-2 minutes on each side, until browned. Remove from heat and let cool slightly.

4. Brush each fillet with Dijon mustard, then wrap them in prosciutto slices.

5. In the same skillet, melt butter over medium heat. Add chopped mushrooms, minced garlic, and chopped fresh thyme. Cook until the mushrooms release their moisture and the mixture is dry. Remove from heat and let cool.

6. Roll out the keto puff pastry dough on a floured surface into a large rectangle, about 1/4-inch thick.

7. Spread the mushroom mixture evenly over the puff pastry, leaving a border around the edges.

8. Place the wrapped fillets on top of the mushroom mixture.

9. Fold the puff pastry over the fillets, sealing the edges and trimming any excess dough.

10. Brush the pastry with beaten egg for a golden finish.

11. Transfer the beef Wellington to a baking sheet lined with parchment paper.

12. Bake in the preheated oven for 25-30 minutes, or until the pastry is golden brown and the beef is cooked to your desired level of doneness.

13. Let the beef Wellington rest for a few minutes before slicing and serving.

Nutritional values: (per serving)

- Calories: 600

- Fat: 45g

- Carbohydrates: 8g

- Protein: 40g

Conclusion

As we reach the culmination of our exploration into the carnivore diet and the power of animal-based nutrition, it is evident that we stand at the threshold of a profound paradigm shift in our understanding of optimal health and wellness. Throughout this journey, we have uncovered the ancient wisdom of our ancestors, rediscovered the nutrient-rich bounty of the natural world, and embraced the transformative potential of the carnivore lifestyle.

From the foundational principles of the carnivore diet to the scientific evidence supporting its efficacy, we have witnessed the undeniable impact of animal-based nutrition on our physical, mental, and emotional well-being. We have heard the inspiring stories of individuals who have reclaimed their health, overcome chronic conditions, and achieved newfound vitality through the power of animal foods.

But our journey does not end here. As we look to the future, we are called to continue our exploration, to remain open-minded and curious, and to embrace the evolving landscape of nutrition and wellness. The carnivore diet is not a one-size-fits-all solution, but rather a framework that invites us to customize and adapt our approach based on individual needs and goals.

As we navigate the complexities of modern life, let us remember the timeless wisdom of our ancestors and the innate connection between humans and the natural world. Let us honor the sacred bond between humans and animals, recognizing the vital role that animal foods play in nourishing our bodies, minds, and spirits.

In closing, I invite you to carry forward the knowledge and insights gained from this journey, to continue exploring the power of animal-based nutrition, and to embrace the carnivore lifestyle as a pathway to optimal health, vitality, and well-being. Together, let us unlock the full potential of our bodies and

minds, and embark on a lifelong journey of

growth, transformation, and abundance.